A Global Response to Elder Abuse and Neglect:

Building Primary Health Care Capacity to Deal with the Problem Worldwide: Main Report

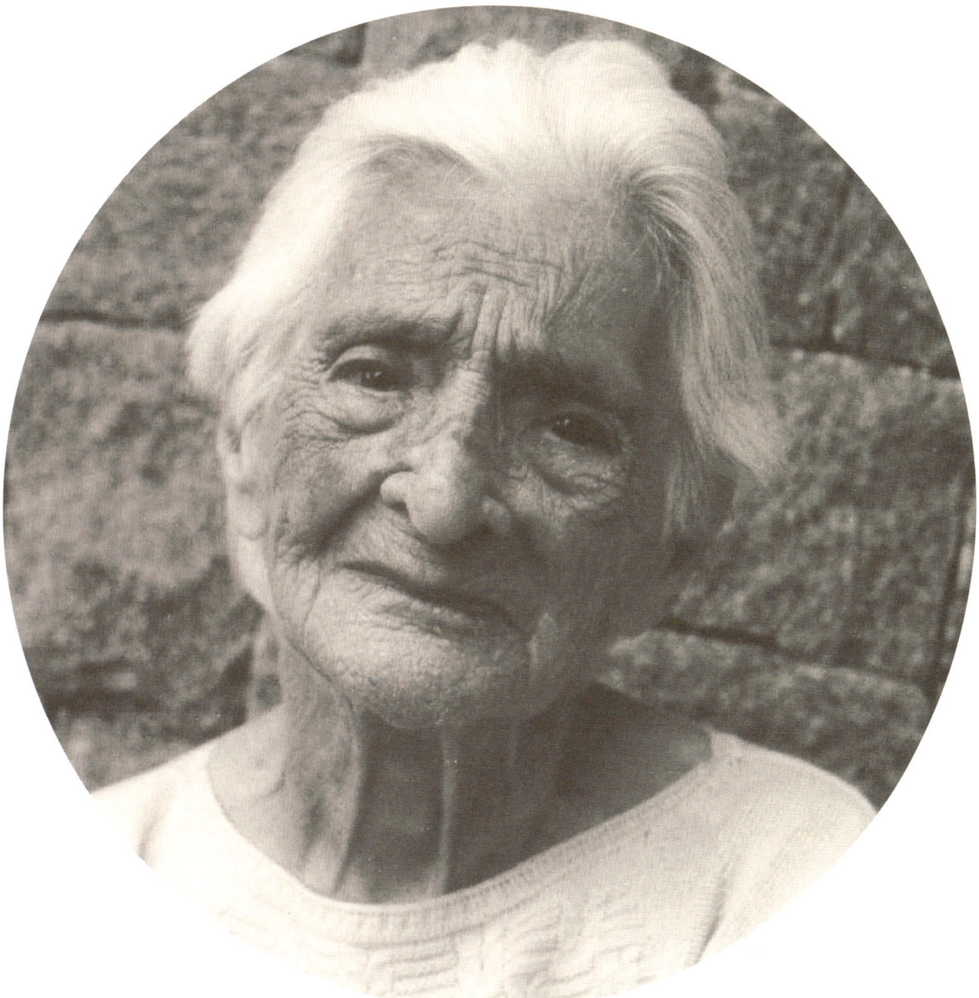

World Health Organization

WHO Library Cataloguing-in-Publication Data

A global response to elder abuse and neglect : building primary health care capacity to deal with the problem worldwide : main report.

1.Elder abuse – diagnosis. 2.Elder abuse - prevention and control. 3.Mass screening. 4.Primary health care. I.World Health Organization. II.Université de Genève. Centre interfacultaire de gérontologie.

ISBN 978 92 4 156358 1 (NLM classification: WT 30)

Printed in France

Acknowledgements

This publication results from the joint research programme "A Global Response to Elder Abuse and Neglect: Building Primary Health Care Capacity to Deal with the Problem Worldwide" undertaken by the World Health Organization Ageing and Life Course Department (WHO/ALC) and the Center for Interdisciplinary Gerontology at the University of Geneva (CIG-UNIGE). The project was initiated and supervised by Dr Alexandre Kalache, Director of the WHO Ageing and Life Course Department, and by Professor Charles-Henri Rapin, Adjunct Professor at the University of Geneva/University Hospital of Geneva. Ms Karina Kaindl coordinated the project and wrote this report under the direction of the project supervisors. Silvia Perel-Levin (ALC) served as first project manager and provided initial technical advice for this document.

The project received technical and financial support from the Department of Noncommunicable and Chronic Diseases and the Family and Community Health Cluster of WHO and from CIG-UNIGE. Gratefully acknowledged are the cooperation and support of the Ministry of Social Welfare and Labour (IMSERSO) and Spanish Society of Geriatrics and Gerontology (SEGG), which provided funding for the research in Spain and for the costs that emerged for the translation into Spanish, and of the Department for Victorian Communities, which organized, carried out and funded the research in Australia.

The study coordinators wish to warmly thank their research partners from Montreal who provided the set of questions and the Social Work Evaluation Form originally devised and piloted by them, both tested within this project.[1] The Montreal team has also generously provided the focus group research protocol used locally and their expert advice. Special thanks are due to the older people, primary health care (PHC) professionals and social workers who took part in the national studies of the participating countries. Gratefully acknowledged are the technical contributions of our research experts, evaluators, country coordinators, focus group facilitators and reviewers.[2]

The generous financial support for the completion of this study and publication of this report was provided by the Geneva International Academic Network (GIAN; http://www.ruig-gian.org). GIAN is an international research network founded by the University of Geneva, the Graduate Institute of International Studies (GIIS) and the Graduate Institute of Development Studies (GIDS). Its main objective is to create synergies among various entities, principally academic institutions and international organizations, through support for policy-relevant research in the service of peace and justice.

1. The team consists of researchers Mark Yaffe (McGill University and St Mary's Hospital Centre), Maxine Lithwick (CSSS René-Cassin) and Christina Wolfson (McGill University and Sir Mortimer B. Davis Jewish General Hospital).
2. A list of the research experts, evaluators and country coordinators can be found on pp. 35–36.

Table of contents

Preface

United Nations estimates indicate that by 2025 the number of older people[3] will double from the current 600 million to 1.2 billion. Of the one million people who reach their sixtieth birthday each month, 80% are in the developing world. Although the proportion of older people out of the total population is higher in developed countries, the percentage increase of the elderly population is much greater in the developing world (UN Population Division, 2004). Furthermore, rapid ageing in developing countries is taking place in the context of fast social change, such as urbanization, increased participation of women in the workplace, industrialization and prevailing poverty. Although elder abuse is not a new phenomenon, the speed of population ageing worldwide, in the context of such profound societal changes, inevitably will lead to an increase in its incidence and prevalence.

Until very recently, elder abuse, the mistreatment of older people, was a social problem hidden from public view and mostly regarded as a private matter. However, elder abuse is a manifestation of the timeless phenomenon of interpersonal violence. Child and partner (mainly female) abuse were the first to emerge and were both seen as mostly family (domestic) violence issues. Public awareness towards child abuse and violence against women gained prominence only once studies in the last quarter of the twentieth century provided evidence of their magnitude. As a consequence, interpersonal violence was then framed only within age-specific compartments. Apart from other parameters that try to explain victimization in different population groups, ageing may trigger an additional risk of abuse due to the increased dependence on others, social isolation and frailty that accompany it. Moreover, older men and women come from generations that avoided discussing private issues. As a result, elder abuse continues to be a taboo, mostly underestimated and ignored by societies across the world.

Evidence is accumulating, however, to indicate that elder abuse, which includes the pervasive issue of neglect, is an important public health and societal problem that manifests itself in both developing and developed countries. As such, it demands a global orchestrated response. From a health and social perspective, unless the primary health care (PHC) and social services sectors are well equipped to identify and deal with the problem, elder abuse will continue to be underdiagnosed and overlooked.

WHO/ALC and CIG-UNIGE, with partners from all continents, conducted this study in order to develop a strategy to prevent elder abuse within the PHC context. The study consisted of a qualitative research project in eight participating countries focused on testing questions originally devised by researchers in Montreal. These questions were aimed at raising awareness among PHC professionals of the issue of elder abuse.

3. Throughout this text "older people" are generally defined as people who are over 65 years old, but in this definition here "older people" are defined as those over 60 years old.

Abbreviations

ALC	Ageing and Life Course Programme/World Health Organization
CIG	Center for Interdisciplinary Gerontology
CSSS	Centre de Santé et de Services Sociaux
EASI	Elder Abuse Suspicion Index
GIAN	Geneva International Academic Network
GIDS	Graduate Institute of Development Studies
GIIS	Graduate Institute of International Studies
HAI	HelpAge International
HUG	Hôpitaux Universitaires de Genève (University Hospital of Geneva)
IMSERSO	Ministry of Social Welfare and Labour (Spain)
INPEA	International Network for the Prevention of Elder Abuse
MIPAA	Madrid International Plan of Action on Ageing
NGO	nongovernmental organization
PAHO	Pan-American Health Organization
PHC	primary health care
Poliger	Policlinique de Gériatrie des Hôpitaux Universitaires de Genève (Geriatric Policlinic of the University Hospital of Geneva)
SEGG	Spanish Society of Geriatrics and Gerontology
SWEF	Social Work Evaluation Form
UNIGE	University of Geneva
WHO	World Health Organization

1 Executive summary

The World Health Organization (WHO) and the Center for Interdisciplinary Gerontology/University of Geneva (CIG/UNIGE), in association with institutions in eight countries (Australia, Brazil, Chile, Costa Rica, Kenya, Singapore, Spain and Switzerland), formed a joint research programme aimed at tackling a substantial and yet hidden social problem: elder abuse and neglect. The foundations of the study were provided by the ground-breaking work conducted by a multidisciplinary and inter-institutional team from Montreal.

The project objectives are:

- To develop and validate a reliable instrument applicable in different geographical and cultural contexts in order to increase awareness among PHC professionals to the problem of elder abuse and neglect.
- To build the capacity of PHC workers to deal with elder abuse and neglect through evidence-based education for the development of prevention strategies.

The original project outline comprised the development and validation of a universal routine screening tool to facilitate the detection of elder abuse and neglect among PHC professionals. Consultations with experts and advisers during the initiation phase of the project, however, have indicated that it is critical to apply the concept of an elder abuse screening tool in the field of PHC; elder abuse involves psychosocial moments of stress not only for the patients but also for the PHC professionals, who are currently not equipped well enough with follow-up strategies. It was considered more appropriate to ultimately develop a tool that helps raise awareness about the issue of elder mistreatment among the PHC professionals and sensitizes them in dealing with potential abuse cases. Therefore, the goal of the WHO-CIG study is to provide an instrument to detect suspicions of elder abuse modelled on the Elder Abuse Suspicion Index (EASI), a questionnaire previously developed and tested in Montreal.

Elder abuse and its detection are challenging and highly sensitive issues that need a linguistically and culturally specified approach and vocabulary. Consequently, the creation of a "universal" tool implies global testing. The first step was the qualitative testing of a set of questions, which led to the Montreal EASI, in the eight participating countries mentioned above. Further action such as the piloting of the tool in clinical settings and the expansion of the range of participating countries will be the basis for future studies.

The results of the study confirm that in the opinion of the older people involved and, in particular, of the PHC professionals, the provision of a short instrument covering key dimensions of elder abuse might be a critical step in preventing and detecting such abuse. According to such results, however, a universal instrument applicable to all cultural and geographical contexts has not yet been developed; the appropriateness of its content and wording vary, depending on the setting. Nevertheless, the study participants believe that it is essential to equip PHC professionals with a set of questions to serve as a starting point in raising awareness about elder abuse.

Résumé d'orientation

L'Organisation mondiale de la Santé (OMS) et le Centre interfacultaire de Gérontologie de l'Université de Genève (CIG-UNIGE), en association avec des institutions de huit pays (Australie, Brésil, Chili, Costa Rica, Kenya, Singapour, Espagne et Suisse) ont formé un programme de recherche conjoint visant à répondre à un problème social de grande importance qui reste cependant caché, celui de la maltraitance des personnes âgées. Cette étude se base sur le travail novateur mené par une équipe multidisciplinaire et interinstitutionnelle de Montréal[4].

Les objectifs du projet sont les suivants:

- Développer et valider un instrument fiable, applicable aux différents contextes géographiques et culturels visant à améliorer la sensibilisation des agents de soins primaires de santé à la maltraitance des personnes âgées.
- Fournir aux agents de soins primaires de santé les moyens de traiter ce problème grâce à une formation concrète axée sur l'acquisition et la mise au point de stratégies de prévention.

Le projet original s'articule autour du développement et de la validation d'un outil universel de dépistage permettant aux agents de soins primaires de santé de détecter plus facilement la maltraitance et la négligence envers les personnes âgées. Cependant, les experts et les conseillers consultés durant la phase initiale du projet ont souligné la difficulté de mettre en place, lors de soins primaires de santé, un outil de dépistage de la maltraitance des personnes âgées en raison du stress – occasionné par la situation de soins – ressenti tant par les patients que par les professionnels de santé qui ne disposent actuellement pas de stratégies de suivi adéquates. Il a été jugé plus opportun de se focaliser sur le développement d'un outil qui aide les professionnels de la santé à mieux prendre conscience de la maltraitance chez les personnes âgées et à les sensibiliser au traitement de cas potentiels d'abus. Par conséquent, l'objectif de l'étude de l'OMS-CIG est de procurer un instrument visant à identifier les cas de

4. L'équipe est composée de trois chercheurs: Mark Yaffe (Université McGill et Centre Hospitalier de St. Mary), Maxine Lithwick (CSSS René-Cassin), et Christina Wolfson (Université McGill et Sir Mortimer B. Davis Hôpital Général Juif).

suspicion de maltraitance à l'encontre des personnes âgées, basé sur le Elder Abuse Suspicion Index (EASI) dont le questionnaire a été précédemment développé et testé à Montréal.

Détecter la maltraitance des personnes âgées est un problème délicat et difficile à résoudre, nécessitant une approche et un vocabulaire spécifiques, définis culturellement et linguistiquement. Par conséquent, la création d'un outil "universel" implique des tests globaux. Il était nécessaire, qu'en premier lieu, nous testions qualitativement l'ensemble des questions – celles qui ont mené au EASI – dans les huit pays participants au projet, mentionnés ci-dessus. Nous projetons de tester cet outil dans un cadre clinique et d'élargir l'éventail des pays participants dans le cadre de futures études.

Les résultats de l'étude, basés sur l'opinion des personnes âgées et plus particulièrement sur celle des professionnels de la santé, confirment que la construction d'un questionnaire court, recouvrant les dimensions essentielles de la maltraitance envers les personnes âgés, pourrait constituer une étape décisive pour mieux la prévenir et la détecter. Cependant, selon ces résultats, la construction d'un outil universel, applicable à tous les contextes culturels et géographiques, n'a pas encore abouti; la justesse de son contenu et sa formulation varient selon le contexte considéré. Néanmoins, les participants à l'étude ont indiqué qu'il était essentiel que les agents de soins primaires de santé disposent d'un questionnaire leur servant de point de départ pour les sensibiliser à la maltraitance chez les personnes âgées.

Resumen técnico

La Organización Mundial de la Salud y el Centro de Gerontología Interdisciplinaria/ Universidad de Ginebra, en asociación con instituciones de ocho países (Australia, Brasil, Chile, Costa Rica, Kenia, Singapur, España y Suiza), han llevado a cabo un trabajo de investigación conjunto cuyo objetivo era abordar un problema social sustancial, todavía bastante oculto: el maltrato y la negligencia hacia las personas mayores. Las bases para la realización de este estudio fueron proporcionadas gracias al trabajo de un equipo multidisciplinar e interinstitucional de Montreal[5].

Los objetivos del proyecto son:

- Desarrollar y validar un instrumento fiable aplicable en diferentes contextos geográficos y culturales con el objetivo de incrementar la concienciación entre los profesionales de Atención Primaria sobre el maltrato y la negligencia hacia las personas mayores.
- Capacitar a los trabajadores de Atención Primaria para el abordaje del maltrato y la negligencia hacia las personas mayores a través de la educación basada en la evidencia para el desarrollo de estrategias de prevención.

El proyecto original consistía en el desarrollo y validación de un instrumento universal y rutinario de cribado que facilitara la detección del maltrato y la negligencia hacia las personas mayores entre los profesionales de Atención Primaria. Sin embargo, las consultas con expertos y asesores durante la fase inicial del proyecto señalaron lo crítico de aplicar el concepto de un instrumento de cribado para el maltrato a mayores en el campo de la Atención Primaria, ya que incluye momentos de estrés psicosocial no sólo para los pacientes sino también para los profesionales de Atención Primaria, quienes actualmente no están dotados adecuadamente con estrategias de seguimiento. Se consideró, por tanto, más apropiado desarrollar un instrumento que ayudara a incrementar la concienciación sobre el tema del maltrato hacia personas mayores entre los profesionales de Atención primaria y los sensibilizara para el abordaje de posibles casos de maltrato. Por tanto el objetivo del estudio de la OMS-CIG es

5. El equipo consiste en los investigadores Mark Yaffe (McGill University and St. Mary's Hospital Centre), Maxine Lithwick (CSSS René-Cassin), and Christina Wolfson (McGill University and Sir Mortimer B. Davis Jewish General Hospital).

proporcionar un instrumento para detectar la sospecha de maltrato hacia las personas mayores basado en el Índice de Sospecha de Maltrato hacia Personas Mayores (Elder Abuse Suspicion Index, EASI), desarrollado y probado previamente en Montreal.

El maltrato hacia las personas mayores y su detección son cuestiones que exigen mucho esfuerzo y son muy delicadas, por tanto, necesitan un enfoque y un vocabulario específico tanto a nivel lingüístico como cultural. De manera que, la creación de un instrumento "universal" requiere un análisis global. Se consideró que un primer paso debía ser el análisis cualitativo de una serie de preguntas, las utilizadas en el EASI de Montreal, en los ocho países participantes mencionados anteriormente. Una acción adicional, que se llevará a cabo en estudios posteriores, es el pilotaje del instrumento en ámbitos clínicos y el aumento del número de países participantes.

Los resultados del análisis cualitativo de las preguntas confirman que, según la opinión de las personas mayores que participaron y, en particular de los profesionales de Atención Primaria, tener un instrumento breve que cubra las dimensiones principales del maltrato a mayores podría ser un paso crítico para su prevención y detección. Sin embargo, de acuerdo con tales resultados, el desarrollo de un instrumento universal aplicable en todos los contextos culturales y geográficos todavía no se ha alcanzado; la adecuación de su contenido y formulación varía en función del ámbito. No obstante, los participantes en el estudio indicaron que creían que esto era esencial para equipar a los profesionales de Atención Primaria con una serie de preguntas las cuales pueden servir como punto de partida para incrementar la concienciación sobre el maltrato hacia personas mayores.

1 Research background

1.1 What is elder abuse and neglect?

The WHO-CIG adopted the definition developed by Action on Elder Abuse (UK)[6] in 1995:

"Elder abuse is a single or repeated act or lack of appropriate action, occurring within any relationship where there is an expectation of trust which causes harm or distress to an older person."

Elder abuse has serious consequences for the health and well-being of older people and can be of various forms: physical, verbal, psychological/emotional, sexual and financial. It can also simply reflect intentional or unintentional neglect. Abuse and neglect are culturally defined phenomena that reflect distinctions between values, standards and unacceptable interpersonal behaviours.

Like any other form of abuse, elder abuse is a violation of human rights and a significant cause of injury, illness, lost productivity, isolation and despair. The study "Missing voices: views of older persons on elder abuse" (WHO/INPEA, 2002a) indicated that older people perceive abuse under three broad areas: neglect (isolation, abandonment and social exclusion), violation (of human, legal and medical rights) and deprivation (of choices, decisions, status, finances and respect).

Modernization, industrialization, an ageing population, urbanization and an increase in the number of women in the workforce may explain increased reports of elder abuse. Prevalence rates/estimates exist only in selected countries and have so far generally been restricted to a few developed nations. Where there are prevalence studies on elder abuse, rates range between 1% and 35% (Pillemer & Finkelhor, 1988; Ruiz Sanmartín et al., 2001; Yan & Tang, 2001), depending on definitions and survey and sample methods. These figures, however, may represent only the tip of the iceberg, and some experts believe that elder abuse is underreported by as much as 80%. Estimates of the number of elder abuse cases reported range from 1 in 15 cases to 1 in 6 cases. These low rates may be due to the isolation of older people, the lack of uniform reporting laws and the general resistance of people – including professionals – to report suspected cases of elder abuse and neglect. In developing countries, although there is no systematic collection of statistics or prevalence studies, crime and social welfare records, journalistic reports and small-scale studies provide evidence that abuse, neglect and financial exploitation of older people appear to be widely prevalent.

6. See also http://www.elderabuse.org.uk/Mainpages/Questions.htm

1.2 Preliminary work

The WHO-CIG joint programme responds to the recommendations of the Madrid International Plan of Action on Ageing (MIPAA) (UN, 2002), the principal outcome of the World Assembly on Ageing, which took place in Madrid, April 2002. The MIPAA is based on the United Nations Principles for Older Persons adopted in 1991 by the United Nations General Assembly under the slogan "To add life to the years that have been added to life", which encapsulates the needed effort towards a just society for all ages. The MIPAA has several implications that address the issue of elder abuse. It calls for changes in attitudes, policies and practices at all levels and in all sectors in order to ensure that people everywhere are able to age with security and dignity, as citizens with full rights. Furthermore, the MIPAA recognizes the universality of the problem of elder abuse. Although the MIPAA points out that the process of ageing brings with it a declining ability to heal and that the impact of trauma may be worsened because shame and fear may result in reluctance to seek help, it also emphasizes that elder abuse is often not solely of a physical form. In this respect, the MIPAA sets out as objectives the elimination of all forms of neglect, abuse and violence directed at older people and the creation of supporting services that address elder abuse.

The MIPAA delineates three priority directions: older people and development; advancing health and well-being into old age; and ensuring enabling and supportive environments. Each of these directions has major implications in the needed global effort to fight elder abuse. More specifically, the MIPAA strongly recommended more emphasis on the prevention and management of elder abuse through the adoption of multisectorial, interdisciplinary community-based approaches to eliminate all forms of neglect, abuse and violence. Furthermore, the MIPAA states that there is an urgent need worldwide to expand educational opportunities in the field of geriatrics and gerontology for all health professionals who work with older people and to expand educational programmes on older people's health for professionals in the social services sector. Informal caregivers also need access to information and basic training on the care of older people. This goes together with the encouragement of health and social services professionals to report suspected elder abuse as well as with the demand on health and social services professionals to inform older people suspected of suffering abuse about the protection and support that can be offered.

WHO has recognized the need to establish a global strategy for the prevention of the mistreatment of older people. The WHO Ageing and Life Course Programme (ALC) has been working in the field of elder abuse since early 2000. In 2002 the results of a multicentric study conducted by ALC in collaboration with the International Network for the Prevention of Elder Abuse (INPEA), HelpAge International (HAI) and partners from academic institutions in a range of countries as well as nongovernmental organizations (NGOs) representing grass-roots organizations over the previous two years were published. The study focused on the views and perceptions of older people and PHC workers of elder abuse through focus groups held in eight countries (Argentina, Austria, Brazil, Canada, India, Kenya, Lebanon and Sweden). The resulting publication "Missing voices: views of older persons on elder abuse" (WHO/INPEA, 2002a) was considered a milestone in the field and has led to the development of further research. In November 2002, WHO, together with INPEA and academic partners, launched "The Toronto declaration for the global prevention of elder abuse" (WHO/INPEA, 2002b) at the Ontario Elder Abuse Conference. This declaration is a call for action aimed at preventing elder abuse worldwide.

Over the years, the Center for Interdisciplinary Gerontology at the University of Geneva (CIG-UNIGE) and the Policlinique de Gériatrie des Hôpitaux Universitaires de Genève (POLIGER-HUG) have undertaken important research on elder abuse, such as the development of screening tools and training courses for social and health workers. This seminal work has been conducted in partnership with the Internet network Vieillir en Liberté (RIFVEL; http://www.fep.umontreal.ca/violence/) for the exchange of information among French-speaking communities and in close relationship with local grassroots organizations. Moreover, in 2004, POLIGER organized in collaboration with CIG and a variety of other institutions the international colloquium HEATWAVE 2004. Specialists from various domains discussed and presented their perspectives, interpretations and advice on elder abuse, with the purpose of coming up with a simple plan of action for future heatwaves in order to draw a lesson from summer 2003, when approximately 40 000 older people died in Europe due to neglect and inappropriate care.

The cooperation between existing public health, social, medical and legal activities and systems needs to be improved, as they depend on each other for the prevention, detection and reduction of elder abuse. As a response, in January 2004, the WHO-CIG project "A Global Response to Elder Abuse and Neglect: Building Primary Health Care Capacity to Deal with the Problem Worldwide" was initiated.

1.3 Elder abuse and neglect and the role of PHC professionals

Since the appearance of the term "granny battering" in 1975 (Baker, 1975), physicians have generally been slow to react towards the issue of elder abuse and neglect. The paucity of research in this area has been matched by limited awareness among PHC professionals. Research on assessing interpersonal violence in adolescents, young adults and women is far more advanced than that on elder abuse and neglect, which are recognized as problems in need of attention over a longer period of time.

Perceptions are changing, reflecting results from studies in many countries. [7] Elder abuse is starting to be recognized as a serious social and (public) health issue. The occurrence and severity of elder mistreatment are likely to increase markedly over the coming decades, as the population ages, as caregiving responsibilities and relationships change and as increasing numbers of older people require long-term care.

The United States National Research Council (National Research Council, 2003) recognized that substantial research is needed in order to improve and develop new methods of screening for possible elder mistreatment in a range of clinical settings. Moreover, it strongly recommends systematic studies of reporting practices and the effects of reporting.

Although a comprehensive health-care response is the key to a coordinated community-wide approach to family violence, physicians report only 2% of all reported cases of elder abuse, compared with reports from family members (20%), hospitals (17.3%) and home health aids (9.6%) (Rosenblatt et al., 1996). Even though the detection of elder abuse is an issue in some hospitals, only a few hospitals have appropriate protocols and follow-up guidelines for dealing with the problem (Ahmad & Lachs, 2002; Lachs, 2004).

It is central to understand the nature and value of increased and more refined medical and social surveillance and screening practices and their effect on geographically based elder mistreatment rates. There is no doubt that health-care settings are particularly important. For instance, in the United States, each year approximately 85% of people aged 65 years and older use formal ambulatory care services and 16–20% are hospitalized (National Research Council, 2003). Therefore, physicians need to be able to recognize risk factors and to apply the diagnostic techniques specifically involved in the detection of elder abuse. Many physicians and other PHC professionals, however, are not yet familiar with the definitions, epidemiology, diagnosis and intervention strategies associated with elder abuse, since it is usually not a problem that can be assessed quickly. Nevertheless, emergency rooms, walk-in clinics and family doctors' practices are commonly used by victims of elder abuse. Similarly, the busy primary care office, although hardly the ideal setting for a time-consuming examination, may be the victim's only hope of detection and protection. In each of these settings, an understanding of good assessment practices is necessary for the physician in touch with the potential victim.

The medical profession is only now beginning to turn its attention to research, detection and prevention of elder abuse. Since physicians are in a unique position to detect elder abuse and neglect first-hand, they have a special responsibility to promote greater awareness and effective

7. For example, PubMed delivered 1111 hits for "elder abuse" in February 2006.

interventions for this problem. Physicians cannot tackle elder abuse alone, however. The cooperation between existing public health, social, medical and legal activities and systems needs to be improved, as each depends on the others for detection, for assessment techniques and for the reduction of the occurrence of mistreatment. This is particularly true since a substantial proportion of elder mistreatment episodes appear to occur in frail elder people, who are often least likely to participate in household surveys and who may be difficult to reach due to social isolation. Consultation at the medical practice is sometimes the only regular interaction that older people have outside their home.

1.4 Detecting elder abuse in a PHC setting

Many aspects of elder abuse would appear to make it a condition ideally amenable to traditional public health screening: it is prevalent, it causes morbidity and mortality, and traditionally it would appear that it is often hidden during consultation. But compared with other diseases and conditions, screening for elder abuse is problematic, since some patients are probably not eager to be detected as a potential victim of abuse. Also "true positives" are not well defined by blood tests or consensus criteria used to screen for other conditions and diseases.

Several screening and detection tools for elder abuse have been developed and tested. They have rarely been validated properly for wider use, however. The multiplicity of the tools available reveals the need to develop, through collaborative research, a reliable and simple tool that can be adapted and used in different geographical and cultural settings. This will help to maximize the full understanding and multiple dimensions of the problem.

Screening tools may have several limitations. For instance, some tools are developed only for research purposes, some have low efficiency in clinical settings, the sensitivity and specificity rates of some are not addressed fully, and physicians do not use some because they are too long, their vocabulary is inappropriate or they are designed for home use. The requirements for a detection tool are thus high: It should be practical, be easy and quick to administer, have appropriate and clear wording suitable for different contexts, and show a high sensitivity rate.

Screening tools by themselves are not enough, however. For professionals to be able to use the tools effectively, they need to be aware of the problem and its consequences and to have access to strategies to intervene and achieve positive outcomes for individuals. Among the obstacles physicians must overcome in order to detect elder abuse are a lack of awareness of the problem, insufficient knowledge about how to identify or follow up a potential case of abuse, ethical issues, time constraints, and the victim's possible reluctance to report to physicians. It is crucial, therefore, not only to raise PHC professionals' awareness but also to equip them with sufficient training and intervention strategies enabling them to react appropriately when a person is at risk of being abused or neglected. Above all, they need the confidence to overcome the very real barriers that prevent detection and intervention.

2 The project

2.1 Aims and objectives

Based on the recommended strategies outlined in the "Missing voices" study, the WHO-CIG programme objectives were:

- To develop and validate a reliable instrument applicable in different geographical and cultural contexts in order to increase awareness among the PHC professionals to the problem of elder abuse and neglect.
- To build the capacity of PHC workers to deal with elder abuse and neglect through evidence based education for the development of prevention strategies.

Following the initiation of the project in January 2004, a meeting was held between the project coordinators, the scientific steering committee and members from affiliated organizations. The following recommendations for the study were made:

Although elder abuse is a universal phenomenon that appears in similar forms regardless of its geographical and socioeconomic context, the appropriate responses may vary, depending for instance on local beliefs and values, availability of resources and legal frameworks. However, although the roots of abuse may be very different between societies, cultural norms should not be used as an excuse for mistreatment to occur or to be ignored.

When testing an instrument to detect potential abuse cases, it is crucial to establish basic response mechanisms, otherwise many PHC professionals will remain reluctant to deal with the issue. In addition, standardized training modules that focus on the detection, prevention and management of elder abuse, taking into consideration already existing models, need to be developed.

The "perfect" tool does not exist. Depending on a person's professional background, either an anecdotal or an evidence-based approach is preferred. A balance needs to be found between a scientifically validated and simple tool that is suitable for use by a wide range of PHC professionals and that is also comprehensible by older people. Simplicity is the key to success in ensuring that a tool would be used by PHC professionals. A useful comparison was made to screening for alcohol dependence (e.g. the CAGE[8] tool with four questions; Ewing, 1984). The ultimate goal should be to sensitize medical professionals and raise their awareness about elder abuse and the possibility that it can occur.

General practices and PHC centres seem to be the best locations for the detection of elder abuse within this research proposal. Among PHC professionals, physicians are in the best position to detect abuse, since they are often the first port of call for older people. The difficulty arises from placing another burden on the physician's already full agenda. Nurses may be a valuable alternative, since they often have, depending on the setting, regular contact with patients.

Thus, it was decided that the best option would be to adopt the EASI that had been developed and tested in Canada using focus group discussions to adjust it for cultural and linguistic factors in the eight participating countries.

2.2 The Elder Abuse Suspicion Index

EASI is an instrument that was developed and tested in Montreal by a research team from McGill University, St Mary's Hospital Centre, CSSS René Cassin, and Sir Mortimer B. Davis Jewish General Hospital, with funding from the Canadian Institutes of Health Research. EASI consists of a few copyrighted, brief and direct questions (five questions for the patient and one for the physician) asked in the course of any office physician–patient encounter and formulated in doctor-friendly language. It is readily applicable to cognitively intact seniors (people aged 65 years and older). The EASI was designed not necessarily to detect cases but to raise suspicion of the occurrence of elder abuse in order to justify referral to community experts in elder abuse such as social workers. A secondary aim was to help familiarize family doctors with elder abuse through the repeated use of a simple set of questions about elder abuse. Although EASI cannot guarantee detection of elder abuse or mistreatment, its application already indicates that the doctor is aware of elder abuse and may therefore refer potential cases to social and community services.

The style of the EASI questions and application is along the lines of recommendations found in the relevant literature. The use of explicit, behaviourally specific closed questions, contextually orienting preface statements, and simultaneous assessment of both assault by strangers and abuse by family members/caregivers is appropriate for older adults. Moreover, there are several advantages of in-person interviewing: This permits visual assessment of both the respondent's physical presentation and the respondent's reactions to the questions. Interviews also offer opportunities for nonverbal indications of support. Finally the validity of clinical diagnosis made on the basis of in-person interviews is higher than that of other methods, such as telephone

8. CAGE stands for 'Cut Down, Annoyed, Guilty and Eye Opener'.

surveys, simply because more convergent (or divergent) lines of data are available to in-person interviewers (Acierno et al., 2003).

Compared with other elder abuse screening tools, for example the Hwalek–Sengstock Elder Abuse Screening Test (H-S/EAST)[9], with originally 15 items, the EASI has fewer questions and requires less time to administer (on average two minutes). Furthermore, of the 104 doctors who participated in the Montreal study, 95.8% rated the questions as "very easy" to "somewhat easy", and 70.5% considered the questions to have either some or a big impact on approaching elder abuse (Yaffe et al., 2005).

In the Montreal study, results of the EASI were compared with a Social Work Evaluation Form (SWEF)[10] to validate the tool.[11] This form is a standardized social work assessment to evaluate in greater depth older people at risk of being abused. The form comprises 67 questions and takes an average of 66 minutes to administer. Question 59 was the "gold standard" question to compare and validate the results of the EASI. Within three weeks of the application of EASI by physicians, social workers who participated in the study administered the evaluation form to seniors. The interview took place either at the older person's home or in a safe place to talk that was mutually acceptable to the participant and the social worker. The correlation between the EASI and the SWEF reached a sensitivity rate of 0.44 and a specificity rate of 0.77 (Yaffe et al., 2005).[12]

The findings of this study conducted in Montreal offer excellent groundwork on which to build further research. However, the original EASI project was focused on the reactions from family doctors and older people in the context of a developed urban society. The aim of the WHO-CIG project proposal was to explore the reactions of similar groups in other cultural contexts and to test a set of questions in geographically different settings across the world. Therefore, focus group participants in eight countries commented on the questions used by the Montreal researchers that ultimately led to the development of EASI.[13] This was one step in the process of looking at the validity of the EASI in different cultural and geographical contexts and assessing its acceptance and usefulness among medical doctors and older patients in places other than Canada.

9. See for example http://www.elderabusecenter.org/print_page.cfm?p=riskassessment.cfm
10. This form was developed by the Institute René Cassin.
11. The SWEF can be found in Annex 2.
12. The sensitivity rate indicates the proportion of people with the target disorder who have a positive test result. It is used to assist in assessing and selecting a diagnostic test/sign/symptom. The specificity rate is the equivalent for negative tests and indicates the proportion of people without the target disorder who have a negative test.
13. In the WHO-CIG focus group study, materials from the Montreal EASI project were used according to a memorandum of collaboration between the researchers and WHO-CIG. Questions used in the WHO-CIG focus groups are based on the original EASI focus group protocol (see Annex 1), but the order of the questions was changed and some of the questions were split.

2.3 Research design and methodology

In order to obtain information on specific issues that may vary from one geographical setting to another, focus groups were selected as a method because of their ability to explore beliefs, attitudes and behaviours in a target group. Furthermore, people usually feel comfortable in a focus group discussion because it is a form of communication found naturally in most communities (Hudelson, 1994).

Participants were asked to express their opinions about whether the proposed questions are appropriate, relevant and understandable. Based on these findings, training modules, identification methods and intervention strategies can then be developed or adapted according to local conditions.

The eight participating countries (Australia, Brazil, Chile, Costa Rica, Kenya, Singapore, Spain and Switzerland) were engaged through professional links from WHO and identified according to the following parameters:

- Possibility of collaboration with a local coordinator and a focus group/workshop facilitator.
- Participating countries should cover a wide range of regions. In this case, Africa, South America, Central America, Europe, South-East Asia and the Western Pacific Region were included.
- Follow-up mechanisms should be in place to provide information on local support and service networks in case a piloting phase in clinical settings would follow the qualitative research.

The research design included the conduct of seven focus groups in each country to test the bank of 12 questions that led to the EASI. The groups were split as follows:

- Three groups of older people, broken down further into one group of older women only, one group of older men only, and one group of both older men and women.
- Four groups of PHC professionals.

Each group ideally consisted of six to nine people. The two-hour focus group sessions were tape-recorded, transcribed and analysed, and the findings from each country were summed up in a report.

Furthermore, workshops were organized to test the general reaction of social workers towards the concept of the SWEF and to gather general information on issues of elder abuse, such as local assessment and intervention strategies and culturally specific categories of elder abuse.

In a second workshop, reactions from PHC professionals and social workers were sought to see how useful the Pan American Health Organization (PAHO) guidelines on abuse and neglect were considered to be.[14] This manual could be used as follow-up and intervention strategies for PHC professionals to use concerning the issue of elder abuse and neglect. The comments and reactions gathered in these two workshops were likewise summarized in the country reports.

The WHO-CIG project coordinators provided all the necessary information and documentation for the conduct of the focus groups and workshops, including session outlines and administrative forms. Refreshments or a meal, reimbursement for travel, and information material was offered to the participants. Other forms of remuneration were not included.

In summary, the activities in every participating country included the following:

1. Four focus groups with general practitioners/PHC doctors:

- Expose general practitioners to the bank of 12 questions (brief introduction).
- General practitioners "pilot" the set of questions with a small sample (15–20 patients) to acquire familiarity with the instrument (where possible).[15]
- Focus group discussions with general practitioners on experiences, perceptions and suggestions after the application of the questions.[16]
- Report.

2. Three focus groups with older people:

- Expose older people to the bank of 12 questions (brief introduction).
- Focus group discussions with older people on suggestions and perceptions of the 12 questions.
- Report.

3. Workshop with social workers:

- Introduce social workers to the SWEF.
- Workshop with social workers to seek their views and perceptions on how applicable the evaluation form is within the reality of the country.
- Report.

14. These guidelines are taken from Pan American Health Organization (2002) and can be found in Annex 3.
15. Due to a very tight project schedule, the pre-sampling was possible only in Chile and Spain.
16. Along the lines of the work conducted in Montreal.

4. Mixed workshop on the PAHO manual:

- Introduction of PAHO training model to general practitioners and social workers.
- Focus group discussion following a workshop format on the content of the manual.
- Report.

Since elder abuse is a universal phenomenon, the target of the project was not to apply any social, gender or ethnic discriminations to the study. Certain exclusion criteria are justified, however, with the purpose of protecting participants and for the overall benefit of the study. Therefore, cognitively impaired older people were excluded.

In some countries, it was difficult to find general practitioners or front-line doctors willing to participate in the focus group discussions. In this case, they were replaced by nurses, dentists and geriatricians. The age limit for participants in the focus groups for older people (65 years and older) was lowered in some settings (Singapore) according to the national definition of "older person". "Being literate" was an additional inclusion criterion in Brazil for the focus group discussion held with older people.

The aim of the focus group discussions was to seek the participants' opinions on each of the 12 items by asking:

- How important is this item in detecting elder abuse?
- How do you like the wording of the question? Are there any words that cause problems? What could they be replaced with?
- Is there redundancy within the question?
- Do you think having several issues in one question is too complicated or problematic in any way?
- Is the wording too long – how might it be rephrased?

Furthermore, participants had to choose at the end of the session the five most relevant questions to be included in the final tool.

The project coordinators identified a local coordinator in each participating country who was in direct regular contact with Geneva. This coordinator appointed a local facilitator with a background in qualitative research methodology to organize and conduct the focus groups and workshops, to provide relevant background information, to analyse the data, and to prepare the final country report based on the focus group and workshop sessions. These country reports were translated into English if they were written in a language other than English. Afterwards, they were reviewed and a content analysis was performed in order to obtain feedback on the questions and to discover emerging themes and answers relevant to the identification of elder abuse. Derived from these discussions, the following findings for the tested questions were formulated in order to adapt the instrument and to make it compatible for piloting in the eight participating countries.[17]

17. A summary of each country report can be found in Annex 4.

3 Findings and discussion

3.1 Focus groups with older people

In some countries, the older participants did not clearly understand the purpose of the focus group discussions and the concept of commenting on or discussing the questions (Chile, Kenya). These groups talked about their experiences in relation to each question instead of discussing their content and choosing the five most relevant questions.[18] The groups in Spain discussed a different set of questions and therefore are not taken into account in Table 1.[19]

A number of general issues emerged from the discussions with older people:

- Frail older people's dependence on caregivers could influence their answers. It is therefore crucial to **ask these questions in private.**
- The pressure on general practitioners' time and the cost to the patient would make a **shorter questionnaire** more useful. Lack of training was also a concern.
- An essential issue that was brought up in several discussions was the need for GPs to have **follow-up strategies for a general practitioner** when they identify a person at risk of being abused.

The five preferred questions chosen by the older people in the different settings were Questions 4, 5, 6, 8 and 11 (in order of number of responses):

Table 1. Five preferred questions of older people[20]

Country	Question number											
	1	2	3	4	5	6	7	8	9	10	11	12
Australia				X	X	X		X			X	
Brazil			X	X	X	X	X					
Chile (N/A)												
Costa Rica	X		X	X	X				X			
Kenya (N/A)												
Singapore	X			X	X	X		X			X	
Spain (N/A)												
Switzerland				X	X	X		X			X	

N/A, not applicable.

18. The focus group protocol including the set of 12 questions can be found in Annex 1.
19. See also Summary of report from Spain in Annex 4. Comments that are also applicable to the set of 12 questions are integrated in this chapter.
20. In some countries there were six questions chosen, either because two or three questions were considered equally important or because participants felt that it was necessary to retain six questions instead of five.

The **wording of the questions came across as somewhat stilted and sometimes too "clinical".** The term "prevented" appears to be a poor choice of word: It was suggested that "deprived" (Singapore)[21] and "denied" (Spain) would be better alternatives. Other expressions such as "basic daily needs" (Australia, Brazil, Singapore), "adequate living space" (Costa Rica) and "impeded your free movement" (Australia) appeared to be incomprehensible. "Health aids" and "hearing aids" can be omitted (Costa Rica, Singapore). Some of the questions include too many different ideas and are too wordy (e.g. Question 4). Other questions were too general (Question 10) and could be elaborated better with specific examples. In order to make the questions simple and straightforward, only one idea should be addressed within each item. For example, Question 6 asks about three different things: (i) being taken advantage of, (ii) being prevented from doing things and (iii) interference with being with the people you wanted to be with.

The **questions were, in general, considered to be comprehensive in covering all key areas of elder abuse**. Some forms of abuse, however, such as emotional abuse, neglect (Singapore), deprivation of food and the burden of child care, were considered relevant issues that were not addressed specifically. Also, societal abuse, in the form of "ageism", was a recurring theme. The subtle, and sometimes not so subtle, changes in the way older people are regarded by society as being "less of a person" as they age were an often-expressed concern that was considered by participants to constitute abuse.

Questions 2 and 3, tackling the issues of asking for help and dependence, are good questions, but most older people would find it hard to admit that they need help or depend on somebody.

It was pointed out that it is becoming **less likely that older people have a consistent and close relationship with a doctor** they know; some questions (e.g. Question 12), however, require a trusting relationship between the patient and the doctor and depend on the **doctor's skills to ask the questions in a sensitive way** that would encourage people to trust them.

21. The brackets indicate which country groups are meant or made a specific comment.

Other questions cannot be asked in all cultural contexts. It was a general comment that the **question about sexual abuse** (Question 12) **would be very confrontational** and should not be asked of all people. In Kenya, the issue of sex is considered to be a topic that is too delicate to be discussed with a stranger or even a doctor known to the person. It was suggested that this question should be asked only if there is already some suspicion of sexual abuse.

Depending on the geographical setting, some questions were given more weight and emphasis. The question on **alcohol dependence** was considered much more relevant in Costa Rica and Kenya than in other countries. It was also suggested that drug abuse be included in this question. Question 7, relating to the risk of **financial abuse**, was considered as one of the most important questions by the Brazilian focus group participants. Also in Kenya, financial dependence was identified as a high-risk factor, since almost all households depend on older parent(s) for financial support for food, clothing, fees and medical care. The issue was regarded as less important in other countries, however. The **burden of child** care on older people appears to be an overwhelming concern in Kenya that was not addressed directly by the questions. The Brazilian group of older men and women felt that physicians should not be concerned with the concept of "being taken advantage of", as this was considered a daily issue to which people in Brazil are used.

3.2 Focus groups with PHC professionals

The organization of focus groups with physicians caused difficulties as only a limited number (Australia, Kenya, Singapore) or none (Chile) were willing to participate in the groups. In some countries they were replaced (partly) by nurses (Australia, Chile) or dentists (Kenya).

Some general comments were made throughout the discussions:

- The term **"elder abuse" has a negative connotation** and elicits such fear and anxiety, even among health-care professionals, that there may be a need to look for other terms that can be used to replace it.
- It is essential to **determine whether or not there is a cognitive deterioration in the older patient** before asking such questions, as this questionnaire cannot be used when a patient is cognitively impaired.
- These **questions should not be asked in front of the potential perpetrator**, e.g. a caregiver.

- All of these **questions should be asked in a conversational way** rather than like a questionnaire or checklist. Physicians may not have enough time to ask these questions. Alternatively, in some situations, **nurses could administer the questionnaire**.
- Asking these questions would also **require physical examination** as part of the screening.
- **PHC professionals need to be familiar with the various categories of elder abuse, and follow-up and intervention strategies**, when administering this questionnaire.
- How should a PHC professional react if there is substantiated suspicion of abuse but the potential victim is not willing to denounce the perpetrator or to be referred for **further action**?

The five preferred questions chosen by the PHC professionals in the different settings were Questions 4, 8, 5, 11 and 12:

Table 2. Five preferred questions of PHC professionals

Country	Question number											
	1	2	3	4	5	6	7	8	9	10	11	12
Australia				X		X		X	X		X	X
Brazil				X	X	X		X			X	X
Chile				X	X			X	X		X	
Costa Rica				X	X			X			X	X
Kenya	X			X	X			X				X
Singapore			X	X	X			X			X	
Spain[22]			X	X	X			X			X	
Switzerland				X	X	X		X			X	

Overall, the **questions are considered useful** as the instrument is shorter than other tools and helps in raising awareness. Also, all of the key areas of elder abuse are covered. Issues of loneliness, dependence on others for their basics, being mistreated, being vulnerable at the hands of the powerful, being taken advantage of, overwhelming financial responsibility and being caregivers in their state of fragility are critical issues today that the questions capture. In order to be used effectively, however, it was recommended that the questionnaire **was shortened** and **its wording simplified**.

The **questions appeared to be overly formal and convoluted**. There are a number

22. Only two groups in Spain discussed the bank of twelve questions. The others tested the original EASI (see also the Summary of the report from Spain in Annex 4).

of terms that are too difficult to apply, such as "adequate living space" (Australia, Brazil, Chile, Singapore), "free movement" (Brazil), "unwanted approaches" (Brazil), "health aids" (Chile), "basic daily needs" (Australia, Brazil, Singapore, Spain) "and taking advantage" (Singapore). Other expressions are not specific enough, such as "needed things" (Australia).

Some of the **questions should be separated** as they contain different concepts that are not related to one another. For instance, Question 4 inquires about both basic and secondary needs. Question 5 asks about different emotions ("sad, shamed, fearful, anxious or unhappy") in one sentence. In Question 8, two different issues are addressed: misuse of money and being forced to sign documents. Other questions could be combined, such as Questions 2 and 3, and Questions 11 and 12.

Some words are **difficult to translate** into other languages, e.g. an equivalent for "dependent" (Question 3) does not exist in Mandarin. Generally, it was challenging to translate some of the expressions into Brazilian Portuguese and to translate whole questions into Bahasa Melayu and Mandarin and its dialects.[23]

General remarks looking at the questions as a whole recommended that the **second part of** each **question** (where applicable) **could be omitted** (i.e. "Was this an isolated event or has it occurred more than once?") (Australia, Brazil, Singapore, Spain). It is important, however, to get some idea of whether this is an isolated incident or part of an existing and/or long-standing pattern, even in detecting suspicions of abuse. Furthermore, the **time frame of the questions is not clear:** should the main focus be on recent situations or on events that happened several or many years ago or even within a lifetime? Another suggestion was to add a part asking about the relationship with the perpetrator (Costa Rica, Spain).

Similar to the discussions with older people, it was mentioned that many older people feel uncomfortable when requesting help, either because they want to stay independent or because they are afraid of being rejected. This factor renders it more difficult to identify abuse, as **some people may not answer the questions fully** because they fear repercussions by the perpetrator. A **trusting relationship between the physician and the patient**, where the medical practitioner has prior knowledge of the social or home situation and family relationships of the older patient, is crucial. Moreover, some of the questions (e.g. Question 12) would require several visits to the doctor before they can be asked (Australia, Singapore).

23. For the groups in Singapore, the questions were translated into Mandarin, as the majority of Singaporeans are Chinese and speak not English but Mandarin and its dialects.

Although **sexual abuse** of older people is a category that needs to be included, **it may be detrimental to the well-being of an older person if an untrained person asks about the issue**. Furthermore, there were doubts about whether people would be willing to answer such a direct and delicate question (Costa Rica, Kenya, Spain). Also, the gender dimension was emphasized: It was pointed out that it would be difficult in some countries if a male GP asked an older woman about this issue (Singapore).

The concept of preventing somebody from something needs further clarification (Question 4): At times the necessities of older parents cannot be met because of a lack of financial means and resources (Costa Rica, Singapore), and sometimes life events or health problems curtail the freedoms and choices of older people, such as advice from family or doctors to cease driving a car (Australia). The deprivation of something that is needed by an older person is therefore not necessarily an abuse, although this depends on the definition of need that is being used. Additionally, it should be further specified whether the question refers to a person or an abstract body, for example the community (Spain).

Question 11 was considered ambiguous as it is not clear whether this item refers to **accidental harm** (such as a fall or bruise when transferring someone into a wheelchair or bath) or **intentional harm** (being intentionally rough or violent).

As in the groups with older people, some questions are considered important according to the geographical context they are asked in. Question 9 on alcohol dependence polarized participants. More significance was attached to the question in Australia, Chile and Costa Rica than in other countries. Also **illicit drug-taking and gambling addictions** by caregivers or family members could be added to this item (Australia). However, it was pointed out that drinking too much alcohol should not be considered automatically as a risk factor for elder abuse, but it may be implicated in the development and perpetuation of abusive situations and therefore should act to raise suspicions that abuse exists or has taken place.

Issues that were neglected in the questions were **chemical restraint** (Australia), **threatened physical violence** (Australia), **involvement in decision-making** (Australia), **abandonment** (Costa Rica) and **neglect** (Singapore).

There were only a few comments on the **order** of the questions. In most cases it was suggested to leave the order as it is or to reverse the order of the first few questions.

3.3 Implications of the results for the EASI tool

The country coordinators presented the focus group findings at a meeting where recommendations and conclusions were discussed. Two researchers from the Montreal team also participated in the meeting.

At this meeting, the set of 12 questions was compared with the original EASI[24] (5 questions for the patient and 1 question for the physician). Based on their study results for the 12 questions, the group agreed that the EASI was a good and simple tool that covers all the important abuse categories. Its wording is appropriate for cultural and geographical contexts other than Canada. Question 1 of the EASI is a way of asking older people if **they need help** and to introduce potential **situations of risk**. Question 2 enquires about whether any kind of **deprivation** is taking place. Question 3 covers **psychological and verbal abuse**. Question 4 is about **financial abuse**. Question 5 tackles **physical and sexual abuse**. Question 6a is an **observer question** and Question 6b is a question about privacy and honesty and is only for research purposes. The country findings of the WHO-CIG study indicate that in most focus group discussions, the same questions were chosen as most relevant. The following questions correspond to each other between the two sets of questions:

Question 2 (EASI):

2. Has anyone prevented you from getting food, clothes, medication, glasses, hearing aids or medical care, or from being with people you wanted to be with?

and Question 4 (WHO-CIG focus group questions[25]):

4. Has anyone prevented you from having needed things such as food, medication, clothing, adequate living space, or health aids such as eyeglasses, hearing aids, etc.?

Question 3 (EASI):

3. Have you been upset because someone talked to you in a way that made you feel shamed or threatened?

and Question 5 (WHO-CIG focus group questions):

5. Has anyone close to you unfairly yelled at you, or talked to you in ways that you did not like, or made you feel especially sad, shamed, fearful, anxious, or unhappy – in a way that left you upset for a long time?

24. See pp. 24-25.
25. See also Annex 1.

Question 4 (EASI):

4. Has anyone tried to force you to sign papers or to use your money against your will?

and Question 6 and Question 8 (WHO-CIG focus group questions):

6. Has anyone close to you made you feel that you were being taken advantage of, or prevented you from doing things that were important for your well being, or interfered with you being with the people you wanted to be with?

8. Has anyone that you would trust used or tried to use your money, possessions or property in ways that you did not want, or forced you to sign documents that you did not understand or did not want to sign?

Question 5 (EASI):

5. Has anyone made you afraid, touched you in ways that you did not want, or hurt you physically?

and Question 11 and Question 12 (WHO-CIG focus group questions):

11. Has anyone physically hurt you, for example has hit you, pushed you or has impeded your free movement?

12. To a degree that it upsets you, has anyone touched you in ways you did not like, or made unwanted sexual approaches?

By looking at the EASI questions, a few comments were made. For Question 2 it was mentioned that types of deprivation depend on the cultural context and may need modifications. Furthermore, it was discussed whether "sad" should be included in Question 3, but the project group decided that "sad" is not an emotion that is necessarily associated with situations of abuse. The issue of "neglect" was not addressed adequately in the whole questionnaire. It was also suggested to take out all cases of "Has this happened more than once?". Moreover, a few minor modifications were recommended for the EASI (highlighted below in yellow):

Subject No. ❒❒❒❒❒❒
Doctor No. ❒❒❒

Instructions to patients:

I am now going to move to the research study in which you have agreed to take part. (If there is an accompanying person say to her/him: Since the researchers ask that this be done in private, would you please leave us for a few moments?) If accompanying person does not leave, ask questions anyway, but record below his/her presence...I will now ask about life situations or relationships that may have occurred over the last 12 months. While it may be difficult to do, please try to answer each question with only the words Yes or No.

1. Have you relied on people for any of the following: bathing, dressing, shopping, banking or meals?

❐ Yes ❐ No ❐ Did not answer

If Yes: Have problems been common between those people and you?

❐ Yes ❐ No ❐ Did not answer

2. Has anyone prevented you *or tried to prevent you* from getting food, clothes, medication, glasses, hearing aides or medical care, or from being with people you wanted to be with?

❐ Yes ❐ No ❐ Did not answer

If Yes: Has this happened more than once?

❐ Yes ❐ No ❐ Did not answer

3. Have you been upset because someone talked to you in a way that made you feel shamed or threatened?

❐ Yes ❐ No ❐ Did not answer

If Yes: Has this happened more than once?

❐ Yes ❐ No ❐ Did not answer

4. Has anyone tried to force you to sign papers or to use your money *or your belongings* against your will?

❐ Yes ❐ No ❐ Did not answer

If Yes: Has this happened more than once?

❐ Yes ❐ No ❐ Did not answer

5. Has anyone made you afraid, touched you in ways that you did not want, or hurt you physically?

❐ Yes ❐ No ❐ Did not answer

If Yes: Has this happened more than once?

❐ Yes ❐ No ❐ Did not answer

Doctor: Do not ask this next question to the patient. It is for you only to respond to.

6a. Elder abuse may be associated with findings such as: poor eye contact, withdrawn nature, malnourishment, hygiene issues, cuts, bruises, inappropriate clothing, or medication compliance issues. Did you notice any of these today or within the last 12 months?

❐ Yes ❐ No ❐ Not sure

6b. Doctor: Aside from you and the patient, is anyone else in this room during this questioning?

❐ Yes ❐ No

M.J. Yaffe, MD mark.yaffe@mcgill.ca
M. Lithwick, MSW mlithwick@ssss.gouv.qc.ca
C. Wolfson, PhD tinaw@epid.jgh.mcgill.ca

3.4 Workshop with social workers

There seems to be a general consensus among the participants from the different countries that elder abuse is an important community issue, regardless of the geographical setting. Also **ageism**, in the form of disrespect and disregard of older people, was a theme that was prominent in almost all groups. Nonetheless, **resources and community support are in most cases limited**. Insufficient engagement on behalf of the government affects all participating countries, expressed by prevailing public policies relating to health care, social issues and finance that do not adequately cover or protect older people (Australia, Brazil, Chile, Costa Rica, Kenya, Spain).

The participants discussed culturally specific risk factors for elder abuse and developed the following categories:

- **Family members who are involved in drug dealing** (Brazil).
- **Living in a *favela*** [26] increases the level of vulnerability and isolation by restricting free movement due to the violent environment (Brazil).
- When **witchcraft is suspected** (e.g. among the Kisii of Kenya), it is always older people, rather than young people, who are accused. Many older women are burnt to death by the public, with or without "evidence" (Kenya).
- Unlike in other participating countries, in Kenya the **low number of older people in the total population,** compared with children, leads to a very limited amount of resources being allocated for older people.
- **Access to health care facilities and counselling services** is usually not available for older people living in remote areas as they cannot walk long distances or afford transportation (Costa Rica, Kenya).
- **Discrimination by health insurance funds:** In Kenya, for example, the National Health Insurance Fund accepts membership only below the age of 75 years. In addition, insurance companies demand much higher premiums from older people, thereby locking them out of insurance and putting them at great disadvantage.

There were also mentioned additional abuse categories that arose within the social workers' experience:

- **Decisions were made by family members and not by the older person.**
- Use of **cultural expectations** to justify abusive behaviour.
- The **threat of abuse and intimidation** can be a potent controlling force.
- **Withholding of information** to punish or to take advantage of an older person.

26. Brazilian shanty town.

Policies, protocols and training on family violence exist in all participating countries, but not all institutions have access to guidelines or offer training facilities (Brazil, Chile, Costa Rica, Kenya). Where there is such access, the training offered is often not formal, standardized, systematic or compulsory. Sometimes elder abuse is included in more general training and work protocols (Brazil, Chile, Kenya, Spain). As a consequence, social workers use their professional experience and training from the area of domestic violence of women and children and then adapt it to their work with older people. In Singapore, many decisions concerning older people require the family's consent. Front-line workers are therefore forced to judge situations from the perspective of the families. Furthermore, interprofessional coordination is considered to be the key to intervention but is often in need of improvement or lacking (Spain).

The SWEF was in general regarded by the workshop participants as a very comprehensive and detailed assessment tool.[27] Nevertheless, views about its applicability were mixed. The positive aspects outline the **extensiveness of the form**, covering many factors, questions and themes of which social workers needed to be aware. It could therefore serve as a good prompting tool and a **resource for training purposes**.

The application of this evaluation form in most countries (Australia, Brazil, Costa Rica, Singapore, Spain, Switzerland) was considered to be infeasible. The **length** of the form imposed the main challenge, providing both practical and theoretical difficulties. Another key problem is the perception of the difficulty of getting **honest answers** to many of the questions: Some people minimize their problems in order to avoid trouble. In some countries, social workers' schedules do not include regular home visits and it would therefore not be possible to verify a person's situation at home. A very solid, trusting relationship would be necessary between the person administering the questionnaire and the interviewed person, but such a relationship can be built up only over a period of time. Some of the wording of the form and/or the style of the questions were considered limiting or inapplicable in some countries (Chile, Singapore, Spain, Switzerland).

In addition, the participants expressed their reservations regarding the **application of this form to cognitively impaired people**. The **problem of over-assessing people** was raised, as there are already many assessment tools in use. It was also stressed that **labels such as "abuse" and "neglect" are not often used** by social workers. The goal of social work intervention was seen as improvement of an older person's quality of life and not to accuse and label somebody as "abuser" or "victim".

Further doubts about the applicability of the form concerned intervention issues. **How does the form relate to an intervention plan?** A manual that accompanies the form to assess suspicion and a flowchart

27. Country-specific concerns, suggestions and comments on questions can be found in Annex 4.

adapted to local intervention possibilities was considered to be necessary. The form was viewed as limiting and not providing ample space for the social workers conducting the assessment to explore further. Moreover, possibilities for **intervention often depend on the existing legislation**. Intervention orders, where they exist, are frequently difficult to enforce due to reluctance on the part of the victim to continually report the perpetrator (often somebody close), the general physical vulnerability of the older person and, sometimes, a lack of police understanding and/or capacity to deal with the situation.

The following suggestions were made in order to make the form more applicable:

- The **form could be used over a number of visits** once trust is established.
- The **use of the** form **should be individualized**, depending on the particular circumstances of the older person. Only the parts that are relevant to the social worker's suspicion (e.g. financial abuse) should be used. Its application could be limited to specific areas such as living conditions, family dynamics, addictions of any family members, degree of physical and economic dependence of the older person and social and emotional isolation.
- For a crisis management/intervention situation such as elder abuse, the **questions should be narrowed down** and should focus more on analysing the seriousness, history and frequency of the abuse.
- In order to shorten the form, the **introductory part could be omitted** (up to Question 19), since this information is available from other sources, for example from medical records.

Apart from the form, the participants thought that a number of initiatives were needed. **Preventive measures** should be in place, such as better support for carers, more professionals dealing with the issue, including the police, and a greater awareness in the community of elder abuse and its devastating effects. Older people should have **access to on-call 24-hour support** to report abuse cases or to obtain information. **Greater use of existing legislation relating to sexual abuse, assault and family violence**, which is currently not used or not used sufficiently in elder abuse, is recommended. **Interdisciplinary collaboration involving, for example, general practitioners, social workers and visiting nurses, is crucial** and could be improved by organizing **round tables** for the different stakeholders, including the older people, to share experiences, disseminate information and offer solutions. The teams would hold case meetings and develop individual strategic plans to protect older people in their homes who were at risk or who had taken out intervention orders, where these exist, against an abuser. This would need to be accompanied by regular home visits in order to improve protection for older people.

3.5 Workshop with PHC professionals and social workers

The participants discussed existing assessment and intervention possibilities but also the barriers that can hamper the prevention and detection of elder abuse in the respective countries. [28]

Both professional groups (PHC professionals and social workers) have encountered abused patients but reacted differently. The **social workers appear more willing to get involved** and would want to share with each other their experiences in handling and managing cases of elder abuse. Social workers either interview the abused client and/or find out about the available and appropriate systems of support. General practitioners/**PHC professionals** usually refer the patients to social workers, when they have the necessary information, but they **are more hesitant to become active and often feel powerless**. This reluctance may stem from the lack of time that they have with their patients, from the absence of follow-up strategies or from the expected role and responsibilities attached to each profession. In one setting (Singapore), it emerged that older GPs could relate better than younger physicians to elder abuse.

Several problematic areas were pointed out that impede prevention and intervention efforts. **Policy-makers' awareness of PHC professionals** needs to be increased in all countries. Another issue concerned the **legislation** in some countries (Costa Rica, Kenya, Singapore) that does not cover issues of elder abuse adequately. Brazil has mandatory reporting, but concerns were raised on behalf of the PHC professionals as they were worried about their own safety. Further difficulties in the assessment of elder abuse included a **lack of** (i) training on elder abuse, (ii) interprofessional communication and coordination, (iii) protocols for homogeneous interventions, (iv) specific definitions and terminologies, (v) social support for caregivers and (vi) circulation of information regarding the existing institutional resources.

In order to develop PHC professionals' and social workers' capacities to deal with elder abuse, the following initiatives were suggested:

- **Sensitizing governments** about the issues of elder abuse is one of the priorities. Governmental support would help in engaging PHC professionals, especially physicians.
- General practitioners need to know how to refer patients to other professionals, such as social workers, for the management of suspected cases. The establishment of a local **continuing platform where front-line workers can share information** related to elder abuse is recommended.

28. Similar issues that have already been mentioned in the workshop with the social workers are not repeated in this section.

- Not only should professionals receive training, but also the community should be sensitized and **older people should be informed about their rights**, in particular in relation to abuse, neglect and exploitation.
- **Effective solutions need to include the perpetrator of abuse.**
- The **role of nurses needs to be reviewed**. In some countries, nurses may have more capacity than physicians to deal with elder abuse.

It was considered that a manual with basic information on elder abuse for professionals dealing with the issue was necessary. Participants discussed the usefulness of the PAHO manual[29] and its applicability in their respective countries. Participants agreed that the following points should be modified or added:[30]

1. Definition of elder abuse

a. Sexual abuse, abandonment, neglect and self-neglect should be separate categories.

b. Physical abuse should include "forced medical treatments or intervention".

c. Emotional abuse could be separated from psychological abuse. Emotional abuse focuses more on the outcomes for the victim, such as anxiety, depression, sadness and loneliness; psychological abuse also includes "limiting the resources of a person".

d. The following categories could be added:

   i. Abandonment and institutionalization;

   ii. Family and gendered violence, e.g. continuation of violence against women in later life;

   iii. Decision-making by family members on behalf of the older person when this is not desired by the older person or is not necessary;

   iv. Financial motivation and family greed;

   v. Using fear of abuse, neglect, isolation or abandonment to con trol the older person.

e. The risk indicators are portrayed as an individual rights-based approach. This may not be suitable for societies that place more emphasis on familial rights than on individual rights, such as Singapore.

2. Basis of the diagnostic

a. Under "Risk factors in the family", it was suggested that one main set of missing factors were various types of vulnerability in the older person such as disability, illness or frailty, high care needs and dementia (or other behavioural issues that could trigger abuse). Another area

29. The relevant section of the manual, discussed here, can be found in Annex 3.
30. Numbers refer to specific sections of the PAHO manual.

was failings in caregiver behaviour (e.g. lack of responsibility and greed), history of long-term conflicted relationships and mental illness/personality disorders in the perpetrator and/or the victim.

b. Under "Risk factors in institutions and community homes", staff-to-patient ratios, overcrowding and lack of community and social interactions might also apply.

c. General practitioners are not the "first port of call" in all countries for issues of elder abuse, due to their lack of time and training, e.g. Australia. Therefore, the suggested approach in Diagram 1.1 needs context-specific adaptation.

d. It is assumed in the manual that the older person will have physical symptoms of abuse, which is often not the case.

e. A physician is not necessarily familiar with the patient's history, since some patients change their doctors with a high frequency and the same doctor may not always be available to see an individual.

f. It is implied that conflicts with a family member/caregiver is evident, but stressful relationships are often well hidden or denied.

g. There is no mention of cultural differences or likely needs for translators or interpreters to be present.

h. There is no procedure whereby physicians must ask consent before touching or physically examining older patients; this is especially important in cases of sexual assault.

i. The risk indicators are considered as a useful list, but for physicians it would be adequate to call it a "diagnostic guide", as the indicators were not specific enough. Greater preference was given for a checklist that could be used at the end of the assessment.

j. General practitioners and social workers recommend an adoption of a sociomedical diagnosis in Table 1.2.

3. Basis for treatment

a. The approach of the flowchart is too medicalized. Using the word "treatment" makes elder abuse sound like a disease. The focus should be on removing or lessening the harm caused to the older person by the perpetrators of abuse.

b. In some countries "adult protective services" and mandatory reporting do not exist; nor are there specific intervention orders.

c. Referral options vary from country to country and need to be adapted accordingly within specific contexts.

d. A focus on the rehabilitation and education of the perpetrator often seems to be more appropriate than strategies being directed only at the education of the older person.

e. The term "intervention" can be replaced by "options" or "assistance", as an intervention may seem to remove the agency from the older person.

f. An important issue that was not addressed appropriately in Diagram 1.3 is the need to ensure the victim's safety and that appropriate safety planning takes place for individuals, particularly for patients who do not have the capacity to decide for themselves about accepting services.

g. As for an intervention plan, it was suggested to create a hotline/helpline for PHC professionals. The diagram (1.3) was viewed as slightly inflexible.

5. Suggested reading

a. The literature list needs to be updated.

The participants concluded that the PAHO manual was not considered appropriate for use in Singapore, Spain or Australia for the reasons outlined above.[31] In these three countries, follow-up strategies are already in place that seem to better reflect the country-specific realities. The Brazilian group thought that the manual would be used if it was shorter and adjusted to the Brazilian context – for instance, the flowcharts need some adaptation – as it could raise awareness about abuse and neglect among PHC professionals. In both Costa Rica and Kenya, there was a strong feeling that the PAHO manual's content and issues are appropriate and it could be used readily.

31. The recommendations for the PAHO manual summarized in this section are based mostly on the reports from these three countries. More information can be found in Annex 4.

4 Recommendations and conclusions

Throughout the execution of this project, WHO and CIG embraced an interdisciplinary and interagency approach with the objective of pursuing identification and prevention possibilities for elder abuse in the range of participating countries. The complexity of the research – tackling a highly sensitive topic at a global level and taking into account cultural differences – has shown that multiple steps are necessary to develop appropriate elder abuse identification strategies in response to the call from the Madrid International Plan of Action on Ageing. In particular, it is crucial to include the views of the three main stakeholders: older people, medical doctors and social workers.

The conclusions from the focus group and workshop discussions in the various countries corroborate the findings and recommendations from the EASI study in Montreal:

- An instrument with 12 questions is too long, considering that in most of the participating countries the standard consultation time of a general practitioner is 10–15 minutes or less. A shorter instrument covering all key dimensions of elder abuse has a higher chance of being accepted and applied by PHC professionals.
- Before applying such a questionnaire, it is crucial to determine whether the patient shows significant signs of cognitive deterioration.
- These questions should be asked only when the patient is seen alone.
- It is becoming less likely that an older patient has a consistent and close relationship with a physician who knows the patient well. The questions should therefore be applied by a PHC professional over a few visits in order to establish a sufficient trusting relationship between the patient and the PHC professional.
- In case elder abuse is suspected, it is essential to equip PHC professionals with follow-up mechanisms/referral strategies.

Further points mentioned were:

- Nurses could be important alternatives to physicians in applying such a questionnaire.
- A major challenge of the concept of such a tool arose in the focus group discussions. Some of the questions (e.g. Question 11) are somewhat ambiguous, as it is not clear whether a person was hurt accidentally or unintentionally. A caregiver may need training about appropriate lifting and handling an older person in order to prevent harm or injury occurring in future.

- Another difficulty pointed out by the participants is that some people may find it hard to answer these questions.
- The threat of violence and associated intimidation to an older person is an important issue that is not addressed in the bank of 12 questions.

An entirely accurate comparison of the results from the focus groups with older people and PHC professionals – and additionally across the countries – is difficult to achieve, since the nature of the focus groups conducted and the number of participants varied significantly. The following conclusions can be drawn, however:

- In some countries, such as Singapore, older people and PHC professionals both chose an almost identical set of questions to be retained in the questionnaire, but in other countries the selection differs widely.
- In all the relevant focus groups with older people, Questions 4 and 5 were chosen as the most important, followed by Questions 6, 8 and 11 (with lesser consistency across the countries). The choices made by the PHC professionals were more uniform: Preferences were given mostly to Questions 4, 5, 8, 11 and 12.
- A number of similar points were brought up in both groups (older people and the PHC professionals):
- A trusting relationship between the physician and the patient is important.
- Most older people feel uncomfortable when asking for help.
- Although there was a general agreement that the questionnaire needs to be shortened and the wording simplified, there was no consensus on the length of the questions. On the one hand, some thought that longer questions were more difficult to understand but allow for fewer questions. On the other hand, shorter questions might be more comprehensible but would lead to a longer questionnaire; the more extensive the questionnaire – even if the questions are shorter – the higher the chance of losing the attention of older people.
- The importance of some questions, such as those pertaining to alcohol problems and economic dependence, depends on the geographical and cultural context.
- The question on sexual abuse sparked the biggest controversy. Most older people considered this question too delicate or not relevant enough, whereas PHC professionals thought that it was necessary to include this question.

The main goal of this project was to investigate the feasibility of developing an instrument applicable in different cultural and geographical contexts that could raise PHC professionals' awareness about elder abuse and neglect.

The results show that not all questions are culturally sensitive – for example, the question on sexual abuse – and cannot be asked in all settings. More subtle ways have to be found to address this issue. The results also revealed some discrepancies between the set of questions regarded as suitable by PHC professionals and by older people. Based on the results of this study, we cannot yet recommend the tool to be universally applicable because it cannot conform to cultural sensitivities in all settings. It might be possible, however, to develop a tool that is sufficiently flexible in the core questions used that it could be adapted relatively easily for use in different geographical and cultural contexts.

Nevertheless, it is important to devise a strategy for the hidden and widespread societal phenomenon of elder abuse. The Elder Abuse Suspicion Index together with other assessment techniques – such as an appropriate social work assessment and a manual containing information on prevention, identification and intervention approaches tailored to a variety of local contexts – are important starting points from where future efforts can proceed. We recommend that such initiatives should be developed in all countries across the world. These initiatives should complement efforts aimed at the prevention of abuse and at protecting older people in need in order to address a problem that impacts thousands of older citizens' lives.

5 References

Acierno R et al. Assessing elder victimization: demonstration of a methodology. *Social Psychiatry and Psychiatric Epidemiology*, 2003, 38:644–653.

Ahmad M, Lachs MS. Elder abuse and neglect: what physicians can and should do. *Cleveland Clinic Journal of Medicine*, 2002, 69:801–808.

Baker AA. Granny-battering. *Modern Geriatrics*, 1975, 5:20–24.

Ewing JA. Detecting alcoholism: the CAGE questionnaire. *Journal of the American Medical Association, 1984*, 252:1905–1907.

Hudelson PM. Qualitative research for health programmes. *Geneva, World Health Organization*, 1994.

Jiménez Rodríguez S. *Las Personas Mayores y el Abuso: estudio realizado en el Hospital Nacional de Geriatría Dr. Blanco Cervantes. San José, Costa Rica*, 1998.

Lachs MS. Screening for family violence: what's an evidence-based doctor to do? *Annals of Internal Medicine*, 2004, 140:399–400.

Moya A, Gutiérrez BJ. *Malos Tratos a personas mayores, Guía de actuación. Madrid, IMSERSO/ SEGG*, 2005.

Machado L et al. *Paper presented at the XVI World Congress on Gerontology, Adelaide, Australia*, 1997.

National Research Council. Elder mistreatment: abuse, neglect, and exploitation in an aging America. *Panel to review risk and prevalence of elder abuse and neglect. Washington, DC, The National Academies Press*, 2003.

Pan American Health Organization. *Guía clínica para atención primaria a las personas adultas mayors. Washington, DC, Pan American Health Organization*, 2002.

Pillemer K, Finkelhor D. *The prevalence of elder abuse: a random sample survey. Gerontologist, 1988*, 28:51–57.

Rosenblatt DE, Cho KH, Durance PW. Reporting mistreatment of older adults: the role of physicians. *Journal of the American Geriatrics Society*, 1996, 44:65–70.

Ruiz Sanmartín A et al. Violencia doméstica: prevalencia de sospecha de maltrato a ancianos. *Atención Primaria*, 2001, 27:331–334.

Souza ER et al. La morbilidad hospitalaria por violencia contra ancianos: estudio de la atención de emergencia em dos hospitales públicos de Rio de Janeiro. *Cuadernos Médico Socialies*, 1999, 76:71–82.

Souza ER et al. Extremo da vida sob a mira de violencia: mortalidade de idosos no Estado do Rio de Janeiro. *Gerontologia*, 1998, 6:66–73.

United Nations. Madrid International Plan of Action on Ageing, 2002. New York, NY, United Nations Department of Economic and Social Affairs, 2002 (http://www.un.org/esa/socdev/ageing/waa/a-conf-197-9b.htm), access date: July 2006.

World Health Organization/INPEA. *Missing voices: views of older persons on elder abuse. Geneva, World Health Organization*, 2002a.

World Health Organization/INPEA. The Toronto declaration for the global prevention of elder abuse. *Geneva, World Health Organization*, 2002b.

Yaffe MJ, Lithwick M, Wolfson C. A North American view on elder abuse. Presented at World Health Organization Symposium: WHO Approaches to the Prevention of Elder Abuse, 18th Congress of the International Association of Gerontology. Rio de Janeiro, Brazil, 26–30 June 2005.

Yan E, Tang CSK. Prevalence and psychological impact of Chinese elder abuse. *Journal of Interpersonal Violence*, 2001, 16:1158–1174.

6 Project team

Project coordinators

WHO:

Alexandre Kalache, Head Ageing and Life Course programme, WHO, Family and Community Health, Geneva, Switzerland

CIG-UNIGE/HUG:

Charles-Henri Rapin, Directeur adjoint, Centre Interfacultaire de Gérontologie de l'Université de Genève (CIG-UNIGE) and Médecin chef de service, Programme "Bien Vieillir" des HUG, Geneva, Switzerland

CIG-UNIGE/WHO:

Karina Kaindl, Centre Interfacultaire de Gérontologie de l'Université de Genève (CIG-UNIGE) and Ageing and Life Course programme, WHO, Family and Community Health, Geneva, Switzerland

Silvia Perel Levin and Maria Casares were both part of the project coordination but left the team in December 2004.

Research partners and experts

Mark S. Lachs, Professor of Medicine, Division of Geriatrics and Gerontology, Weill Medical College of Cornell University, New York, NY, United States of America

Maxine Lithwick, Researcher and Social Worker, Centre de santé et de services sociaux de René-Cassin et Notre-Dame-de-Grace/Montréal-Ouest, Montréal, Canada

Mark J. Yaffe, Professor of Family Medicine and Chief, Department of Family Medicine, McGill University, St Mary's Hospital, Montreal, Canada

Collaborating and piloting centres/ country coordinators of the national studies

Australia:

Gordana Marin, Department for Victorian Communities, Office of Senior Victorians, Melbourne, Australia

Brazil:

Laura Machado, InterAge Consulting in Gerontology, Rio de Janeiro, Brazil

Chile:

Pedro Paulo Marin, Catholic University of Chile, WHO Collaborating Centre on Ageing and Health, Santiago, Chile

Costa Rica:

Fernando Morales-Martinez, Hospital Nacional de Geriatría y Gerontología Dr Raul Blanco Cervantes, Calles 18–10, Avenida 8, San Jose, Costa Rica

Kenya:

Ms Amleset Tewodros, HelpAge International, Africa Regional Development Centre, Regional Representative – Africa, Nairobi, Kenya

Singapore:

Susana Concordo, Tsao Foundation, Singapore

Spain:

Mayte Sancho Castiello and Antonio Yuste, Ministry of Social Welfare and Labour/Sociedad Española de Geriatría y Gerontología (IMSERSO/SEGG), Madrid, Spain

Switzerland:

Charles-Henri Rapin, Hôpital de Loëx, Bernex/Geneva, Switzerland

Report evaluators

Terezinha Da Silva, Adviser and Trainer, Legal and Judiciary Training Centre, Maputo, Mozambique

Bridget Penhale, Senior Lecturer, University of Sheffield, Sheffield, United Kingdom of Great Britain and Northern Ireland

Proof-reader

Govind Rangrass, Yale University, Newhaven, CT, United States of America

Annex 1: Focus groups research protocol

Twelve questions for a suspicion index:

Question 1		
Do you usually feel lonely?		
❒ Yes	❒ No	❒ Did not answer

We only have about 5–10 minutes for each question; here is what we would like your thoughts on:

- How important is this item in detecting elder abuse?
- How do you like the wording of the question? Are there any words that cause problems? What could they be replaced with?
- Is there redundancy within the question?
- Do you think having several issues in one question is too complicated or problematic in any way?
- Is the wording too long – how might it be rephrased?

You may now turn the page to Question 2

Question 2

When you need help, do you feel uncomfortable turning to people for help?

❒ Yes ❒ No ❒ Did not answer

- How important is this item in detecting elder abuse?
- How do you like the wording of the question? Are there any words that cause problems? What could they be replaced with?
- Is there redundancy within the question?
- Do you think having several issues in one question is too complicated or problematic in any way?
- Is the wording too long – how might it be rephrased?

You may now turn the page to Question 3

Question 3

Do you depend most of the time on someone for help with your basic daily needs?

❐ Yes ❐ No ❐ Did not answer

If "Yes": Are disagreements common between such people and yourself?

❐ Yes ❐ No ❐ Did not answer

- How important is this item in detecting elder abuse?
- How do you like the wording of the question? Are there any words that cause problems? What could they be replaced with?
- Is there redundancy within the question?
- Do you think having several issues in one question is too complicated or problematic in any way?
- Is the wording too long – how might it be rephrased?

You may now turn the page to Question 4

Question 4

Has anyone prevented you from having needed things such as food, medication, clothing, adequate living space, or health aids such as eyeglasses, hearing aids, etc.?

❐ Yes ❐ No ❐ Did not answer

If "Yes": Was this an isolated event or has it occurred more than once?

❐ Isolated ❐ More than Once

- How important is this item in detecting elder abuse?
- How do you like the wording of the question? Are there any words that cause problems? What could they be replaced with?
- Is there redundancy within the question?
- Do you think having several issues in one question is too complicated or problematic in any way?
- Is the wording too long – how might it be rephrased?

You may now turn the page to Question 5

Question 5

Has anyone close to you unfairly yelled at you, or talked to you in ways that you did not like, or made you feel especially sad, shamed, fearful, anxious, or unhappy – in a way that left you upset for a long time?

❐ Yes ❐ No ❐ Did not answer

If "Yes": Was this an isolated event or has it occurred more than once?

❐ Isolated ❐ More than Once

- How important is this item in detecting elder abuse?
- How do you like the wording of the question? Are there any words that cause problems? What could they be replaced with?
- Is there redundancy within the question?
- Do you think having several issues in one question is too complicated or problematic in any way?
- Is the wording too long – how might it be rephrased?

You may now turn the page to Question 6

Question 6

Has anyone close to you made you feel that you were being taken advantage of, or prevented you from doing things that were important for your well being, or interfered with you being with the people you wanted to be with?

❒ Yes ❒ No ❒ Did not answer

If "Yes": Was this an isolated event or has it occurred more than once?

❒ Isolated ❒ More than Once

- How important is this item in detecting elder abuse?
- How do you like the wording of the question? Are there any words that cause problems? What could they be replaced with?
- Is there redundancy within the question?
- Do you think having several issues in one question is too complicated or problematic in any way?
- Is the wording too long – how might it be rephrased?

You may now turn the page to Question 7

Question 7

Do you have anyone who is financially dependent on you?

❒ Yes ❒ No ❒ Did not answer

- How important is this item in detecting elder abuse?
- How do you like the wording of the question? Are there any words that cause problems? What could they be replaced with?
- Is there redundancy within the question?
- Do you think having several issues in one question is too complicated or problematic in any way?
- Is the wording too long – how might it be rephrased?

You may now turn the page to Question 8

Question 8

Has anyone that you would trust used or tried to use your money, possessions or property in ways that you did not want, or forced you to sign documents that you did not understand or did not want to sign?

❒ Yes ❒ No ❒ Did not answer

If "Yes": Was this an isolated event or has it occurred more than once?

❒ Isolated ❒ More than Once

- How important is this item in detecting elder abuse?
- How do you like the wording of the question? Are there any words that cause problems? What could they be replaced with?
- Is there redundancy within the question?
- Do you think having several issues in one question is too complicated or problematic in any way?
- Is the wording too long – how might it be rephrased?

You may now turn the page to Question 9

Question 9		
Do you live with anyone who drinks alcohol more than you think he/she should?		
❒ Yes	❒ No	❒ Did not answer

- How important is this item in detecting elder abuse?
- How do you like the wording of the question? Are there any words that cause problems? What could they be replaced with?
- Is there redundancy within the question?
- Do you think having several issues in one question is too complicated or problematic in any way?
- Is the wording too long – how might it be rephrased

You may now turn the page to Question 10

Question 10

Do you live with anyone who has a history of mental illness?

❐ Yes ❐ No ❐ Did not answer

- How important is this item in detecting elder abuse?
- How do you like the wording of the question? Are there any words that cause problems? What could they be replaced with?
- Is there redundancy within the question?
- Do you think having several issues in one question is too complicated or problematic in any way?
- Is the wording too long – how might it be rephrased?

You may now turn the page to Question 11

Question 11

Has anyone that you would trust used or tried to use your money, possessions or property in ways that you did not want, or forced you to sign documents that you did not understand or did not want to sign?

❒ Yes ❒ No ❒ Did not answer

If "Yes": Was this an isolated event or has it occurred more than once?

❒ Isolated ❒ More than Once

- How important is this item in detecting elder abuse?
- How do you like the wording of the question? Are there any words that cause problems? What could they be replaced with?
- Is there redundancy within the question?
- Do you think having several issues in one question is too complicated or problematic in any way?
- Is the wording too long – how might it be rephrased?

You may now turn the page to Question 12

Question 12

To a degree that it upsets you, has anyone touched you in ways you did not like, or made unwanted sexual approaches?

❒ Yes ❒ No ❒ Did not answer

If "Yes": Was this an isolated event or has it occurred more than once?

❒ Isolated ❒ More than Once

- How important is this item in detecting elder abuse?
- How do you like the wording of the question? Are there any words that cause problems? What could they be replaced with?
- Is there redundancy within the question?
- Do you think having several issues in one question is too complicated or problematic in any way?
- Is the wording too long – how might it be rephrased?

Suppose the instrument - the ***Elder Abuse Suspicion Index*** - could have only **five questions** - which five would you use? Please circle the five question numbers on the pages with the questions.

Please note:

The questions used above were mostly derived from a research project of the *Centre de santé et de services sociaux de René-Cassin et Notre-Dame-de-Grace* (formerly CLSC René Cassin), *McGill University, and St. Mary's Hospital* in Montreal, funded by the *Canadian Institutes of Health Research*. The intellectual property rights for them rest with the researchers Mark J. Yaffe MD, Maxine Lithwick MSW, Christina Wolfson PhD, and Elizabeth Podnieks RN.

Annex 2: Social work evaluation form

Evaluation Form

Subject No. Evaluator:

Location of interview: Home ❒ Other:

Date Referral Received (yy/mm/dd):

Date of first visit (yy/mm/dd):

Date of second visit (if necessary) (yy/mm/dd):

Subject withdrew from study: Yes ❒ No ❒

Date of withdrawal (yy/mm/dd):

Reason for withdrawal:

SECTION 1: SOCIAL HISTORY: (occupation, marriage, divorce, grief, misfortune, education, immigration, moves, other major events.)

In this section, ask subject to tell you a personal history. During this process, gather information on the above and fill it in below:

1. Sex: M ❐ or F ❐

2. Age: ______

3. Language used during the interview: ______

4. Occupation status (circle all that apply)

1. Retired ______ Type of work? ______

2. Unemployed ______ From what? ______

3. Unable to work for medical reasons ______

4. Employed full time as: ______

5. Employed part-time as: ______

6. Homemaker ______

7. Other: ______

5. Housing

1. Home/apartment ❒
2. Low cost housing/HLM ❒
3. Public housing/LTCF ❒
4. Residence ❒

- Services ❒
- No services ❒

5. Other, please specify: __________

- Are there any difficulties or specific problems that the subject has identified re: housing conditions (salubrity, space, security, satisfaction...)?

  Yes ❒ No ❒ N/A ❒ R/A ❒

If "Yes", explain: __________

6. Country of birth:

If applicable, are you under sponsorship at this time? Yes 0 No 0 N/A 0 R/A 0

If "Yes", what is your relationship to the sponsor?

If the subject is originally from another country, ask questions about any specific events that may have influenced their coming to this country (for example holocaust, war etc): __________

7. Marital Status

1. Married ❐
2. Widowed ❐
3. Separated or divorced ❐
4. Single ❐
5. Common law ❐
   - ▸ different-sex partner ❐
   - ▸ same-sex partner ❐
6. Significant relationship ❐

8. Living Arrangements

Check all that apply:

1. Alone ❐
2. With spouse ❐
3. With common law partner ❐
4. With roommate ❐
5. With child(ren) ❐ How many? ____
6. With grandchild(ren) ❐ How many? ____
7. With other relatives: ____
8. With paid caregiver ❐ ____
9. Other: ____

- **How long have you been in the present arrangement?** ____
- **Is it problematic** (for example: family problem, needs more help, other)? ____

Yes ❐ No ❐ N/A ❐ R/A ❐

If "Yes", explain: ____

____

____

____

9. Describe major life events in the last 12 months: (circle all that apply)

1. None
2. Death
3. Divorce (own or within family) / separation from partner
4. Physical deterioration of subject or the person with whom they live
5. Change in financial status
6. Child or grandchild moving in or out etc.
7. Moving in or out of child's or other relative's home.
8. Other, specify: ______________________________

Explain: ______________________________

____

____

____

____

____

____

____

SECTION 1: FAMILY DYNAMICS

RELATIONSHIP WITH SPOUSE/PARTNER

10. If married, is this a first marriage? *(Apply same questioning if it is a common law commitment or long-term relationship.)*

1. Yes ❐ How long? ______

2. No ❐ How long in current relationship? ______

3. Not applicable ❐ *(Go to question 12)*

4. R/A ❐

11. Most couples acknowledge that there are, from time to time, problems that arise in their relationship. How often would you rate problems in yours, whatever your definition of problem is, using the following:

Never ❐ Occasiona ❐ Often ❐ Very often ❐

Explain: ______

______

______

• **Does your spouse or partner have any specific health problem or emotional problem (include illness, handicap, alcohol or drug or gambling addiction, or mental illness)?**

Yes ❐ No ❐ N/A ❐ R/A ❐

Explain: ______

______

______

If "Yes", describe the impact that it has had on you: ______

______

______

______

If applicable, explore the following questions:

- What is the impact of any difficulties in your relationship?

- If there are any problems within the relationship, for how long has this been occurring?

- Do you describe yourself as being mistreated within this relationship?

Yes ❐ No ❐ N/A ❐ R/A ❐

If "Yes", explain:

Is there any precipitating factor?

Yes ❐ No ❐ N/A ❐ R/A ❐

If "Yes", explain:

- Have things become worse in the last 12 months?

Yes ❐ No ❐ N/A ❐ R/A ❐

If "Yes", explain:

RELATIONSHIP WITH CHILDREN

12. Do you have any children? Yes ❐ No ❐ N/A ❐ R/A ❐

If "No" go to question 14.

If "Yes" how many? ______

Explore the relationship between the subject and the child(ren). If there are any problems, with whom?

Please list relationship: A: ______

B: ______

C: ______

D: ______

Describe any problems: ______

______

______

______

13. Does any child have any specific health problem or emotional problem (include illness, handicap, alcohol or drug or gambling addiction, or mental illness)?

Yes ❐ No ❐ N/A ❐ R/A ❐

If "Yes", explain: ______

______

______

If "Yes", describe the impact that it has had on you: ______

______

______

Does this person live with you? Yes ❐ No ❐ N/A ❐ R/A ❐

RELATIONSHIP WITH GRANDCHILDREN

14. Do you have any grandchildren? Yes ❒ No ❒ N/A ❒ R/A ❒

If "No" go to question 16.

If "Yes" how many? ______

Explore the relationship between the subject and the grandchild(ren). If there are any problems, with whom?

Please list relationship: A: ______

B: ______

C: ______

D: ______

Describe any problems: ______

______

______

______

15. Does any grandchild have any specific health problem or emotional problem (include illness, handicap, alcohol or drug or gambling addiction, or mental illness)?

Yes ❒ No ❒ N/A ❒ R/A ❒

If "Yes", explain: ______

______

______

If "Yes", describe the impact that it has had on you: ______

______

______

Does this person live with you? Yes ❒ No ❒ N/A ❒ R/A ❒

OTHER SIGNIFICANT RELATIONSHIP(S)

16. Do you have any other significant relationships? Yes ❒ No ❒ N/A ❒ R/A ❒

If "No" go to question 18.

Explore the relationship between the subject and the grandchild(ren). If there are any problems, with whom?

Please list relationship: A: ______________________

B: ______________________

C: ______________________

D: ______________________

Describe any problems: ______________________

____

____

____

____

17. Does this person have any specific health problem or emotional problem (include, illness, handicap, alcohol or drug or gambling addiction, or mental illness?

Yes ❒ No ❒ N/A ❒ R/A ❒

If "Yes", explain: ______________________

____

____

If "Yes", describe the impact that it has had on you: ______________________

____

____

Does this person live with you? Yes ❒ No ❒ N/A ❒ R/A ❒

RELATIONSHIP WITH OTHER FAMILY MEMBERS

18. Do you have any other family members with whom there have been problems within the past 12 months? Yes ❐ No ❐ N/A ❐ R/A ❐

If "Yes", what are they? With whom do they occur and how often?

19. Does any other family member have any specific health problem or emotional problem (include illness, handicap, alcohol or drug or gambling addiction, or mental illness)?

Yes ❐ No ❐ N/A ❐ R/A ❐

If "Yes", explain:

If "Yes", describe the impact that it has had on you:

Does this person live with you? Yes ❐ No ❐ N/A ❐ R/A ❐

SECTION 3: QUESTIONS ABOUT ADL'S

DEGREE OF DEPENDENCY

20. Are you:

1. Independent in all ADL's ❐ *Go to question 25*

2. Independent in some ADL's ❐

3. Totally dependent ❐

4. (If applicable) How many people provide assistance? ______

Please list relationship: A: ______

B: ______

C: ______

D: ______

In this section, use the categories listed above and below to help you complete the grid. Subjects may have different caregivers for different tasks.

1. Unaided

2. With assistance from others

3. Totally dependent on others

4. Activity not performed

Activity	Degree of Assistance (1-4)	For each item indicate if the situation is Temporary or Permanent	Who performs the activity? (see A-D, above)	Does the subject live with the caregiver?
Bathing				
Dressing				
Toileting				
Medication Administration				
Housekeeping				
Meal preparation				
Eating				
Shopping				
Transportation				
Mobility				
Other				

21. Ask questions directly to the subject about the type of care that he/she receives and about the relationship with the person who helps him/her:

• **Have there ever been any problems with the type of care you received in the last 12 months?**

Yes ❐ No ❐ N/A ❐ R/A ❐

Describe:

• How frequently would you say that such a problem has occurred?

1. Only once   2. A few times   3. Monthly   4. Weekly

Explain: ____________________

____

____

____

____

• Do you ever feel that you are being deprived of things that you need? (For example: household goods, food, going to doctors, dentures etc.)

Yes ❒ No ❒ N/A ❒ R/A ❒

If "Yes", describe: ____________________

____

____

____

____

• Has this person ever behaved in a way that upset you?

Yes ❒ No ❒ N/A ❒ R/A ❒

• Have there ever been disagreements between you and that person?

Yes ❒ No ❒ N/A ❒ R/A ❒

• Has this person ever handled you roughly?

Yes ❒ No ❒ N/A ❒ R/A ❒

Do you have the food you want?

Yes ❒ No ❒ N/A ❒ R/A ❒

– The quality?   Yes ❒ No ❒ N/A ❒ R/A ❒

– The quantity?   Yes ❒ No ❒ N/A ❒ R/A ❒

- **Has there ever been a day or longer when you did not have sufficient food?**

Yes ❐ No ❐ N/A ❐ R/A ❐

- **Does the person ever refuse to take you shopping?**

Yes ❐ No ❐ N/A ❐ R/A ❐

- **Are you ever made to feel like you are worthless or a burden?**

Yes ❐ No ❐ N/A ❐ R/A ❐

If "Yes", Explain: ____________________

____

____

____

- **Are you ever reluctant or afraid to ask for things that you want or need?**

Yes ❐ No ❐ N/A ❐ R/A ❐

If "Yes", Explain: ____________________

____

____

____

22. Do you have any concerns either in:

1. Feeling secure that help will always be available	Yes ❐	No ❐	N/A ❐	R/A ❐
2. Quality of the care that you receive	Yes ❐	No ❐	N/A ❐	R/A ❐
3. Feeling indebted to the person providing the care	Yes ❐	No ❐	N/A ❐	R/A ❐
4. Other	Yes ❐	No ❐	N/A ❐	R/A ❐

Explain: ____________________

____

____

23. Before you needed any help, were there ever problems in your relationship with any of your caregivers?

Yes ❐ No ❐ N/A ❐ R/A ❐

If "Yes", Explain:

24. Does any caregiver have any specific health problem or emotional problem (include illness, handicap, alcohol or drug or gambling addiction, or mental illness?

Yes ❐ No ❐ N/A ❐ R/A ❐

If "Yes", Explain:

If "Yes", describe the impact that it has had on you:

SECTION 4: PHYSICAL AND MENTAL HEALTH STATUS

25. Do you take any medication? Yes ❒ No ❒ N/A ❒ R/A ❒

26. Do you know what each medication you are taking is for?

Yes ❒ No ❒ N/A ❒ R/A ❒

27. In the last 12 months has your consumption of medication increased?

Yes ❒ No ❒ N/A ❒ R/A ❒

If "Yes", Explain: ____

28. Do you consume alcohol? Yes ❒ No ❒ N/A ❒ R/A ❒

29. In the last 12 months, has your consumption of alcohol increased?

Yes ❒ No ❒ N/A ❒ R/A ❒

30. In the last 12 months have you felt increasingly sad or depressed?

Yes ❒ No ❒ N/A ❒ R/A ❒

If "Yes", Explain: ____

31. In the past 12 months, have you consulted or been referred to a psychologist, social worker, psychiatrist or any other type of therapist?

Yes ❒ No ❒ N/A ❒ R/A ❒

If "Yes", Explain: ____

SECTION 5: LIVING WITH A CARE-RECEIVER

32. Do you live with anyone who is dependent on you?

Yes ❒ No ❒ N/A ❒ R/A ❒

If "No" go to question 34.

If "Yes" what it your relationship to that person? __________

Do you give any of the following types of assistance to the care-receiver?

• Bathing	Yes ❒	No ❒	N/A ❒	R/A ❒
• Dressing	Yes ❒	No ❒	N/A ❒	R/A ❒
• Toileting	Yes ❒	No ❒	N/A ❒	R/A ❒
• Medication administration	Yes ❒	No ❒	N/A ❒	R/A ❒
• Housekeeping	Yes ❒	No ❒	N/A ❒	R/A ❒
• Meal preparation	Yes ❒	No ❒	N/A ❒	R/A ❒
• Eating	Yes ❒	No ❒	N/A ❒	R/A ❒
• Shopping	Yes ❒	No ❒	N/A ❒	R/A ❒
• Transportation	Yes ❒	No ❒	N/A ❒	R/A ❒
• Mobility	Yes ❒	No ❒	N/A ❒	R/A ❒

Other (Describe): __________

• **If "Yes" on any of the above, are there any problems between you and that person?**

Explain: __________

33. Does that person ever threaten or get aggressive with you (whether it is intentional or not)?

Yes ❒ No ❒ N/A ❒ R/A ❒

If "Yes", explain: __________

SECTION 6: FAMILY AND SOCIAL ACTIVITIES

34. Are you involved in social activities? Yes ❒ No ❒ N/A ❒ R/A ❒

If "No", explain:

- **Do you feel that you have enough contact with the children, relatives, friends, neighbors, etc...?**

If "No", explain:

- **Are you involved in family activities as frequently as you would like to be?**

Yes ❒ No ❒ N/A ❒ R/A ❒

- **Are you involved in social activities as frequently as you would like to be?**

Yes ❒ No ❒ N/A ❒ R/A ❒

If "No", explain:

If not, what prevents you?

- Health ❒
- No one to take me ❒
- Not enough availability of the activities that I would like to participate in 0
- Too expensive ❒
- Other ❒

Explain:

- **Has anyone close to you ever prevented you from participating in social activities?**

Yes ❐ No ❐ N/A ❐ R/A ❐

If "Yes", explain: ____________________

SECTION 7A: FINANCIAL DEPENDENCY OF THE SUBJECT

35. What is your perception of your financial situation?

1. Financially self-sufficient ❒

2. Partly self-sufficient ❒

3. Total financial dependence ❒

4. Unknown ❒

Explain: ____________________

____

____

____

36. Are your finances managed by:

1. Self ❒

2. With some assistance ❒

3. Entirely by others ❒

4. Unknown ❒

37. If "Yes" to number 36.2 or 36.3 above, what is your relationship to that person?

1. Spouse / common law partner ❒ ____________________

2. Child(ren) ❒ How many assisting/managing finances? ____________________

3. Grandchild(ren) ❒ How many assisting/managing finances? ____________________

4. Niece / nephew ❒ How many assisting/managing finances? ____________________

5. Friend ❒ How many assisting/managing finances? ____________________

6. Other: ____________________

• **Who is responsible for paying the rent (mortgage or property taxes)?**

• **Have there ever been any problems between you and the person managing the finances?**

Yes ❒ No ❒ N/A ❒ R/A ❒

If "Yes", explain:

38. Does anyone have banking power of attorney?

Yes ❒ No ❒ N/A ❒ R/A ❒

If "Yes", have there ever been any problems with this person?

39. Does anyone have total power of attorney? (notarized)?

Yes ❒ No ❒ N/A ❒ R/A ❒

If "Yes", have there ever been any problems with this person?

40. Have you ever signed any documents that you felt you were forced to sign?

Yes ❒ No ❒ N/A ❒ R/A ❒

If "Yes", what was your relationship to that person who forced you?

What was the outcome of this event?

41. *Ask these questions to subjects who have assistance with managing their finances or have their finances managed by someone else (include those who have given power of attorney):*

- **Are you informed about all financial transactions?**
Yes ❒ No ❒ N/A ❒ R/A ❒

If "No", is this a problem for you? Yes ❒ No ❒ N/A ❒ R/A ❒

- **Have you ever had concerns or suspected that your money was not being managed as you would want?** Yes ❒ No ❒ N/A ❒ R/A ❒

Has this been a problem within the last 12 months? Yes ❒ No ❒ N/A ❒ R/A ❒

- **Are your bank balances what you think that they should be?**
Yes ❒ No ❒ N/A ❒ R/A ❒
If "No", is this a problem that has occurred within the last 12 months?
Yes ❒ No ❒ N/A ❒ R/A ❒

- **Has your money ever been used without your consent?**
Yes ❒ No ❒ N/A ❒ R/A ❒
If "Yes", has this been a problem within the last 12 months?
Yes ❒ No ❒ N/A ❒ R/A ❒

- **Are all your bills being paid regularly?**
Yes ❒ No ❒ N/A ❒ R/A ❒
If "No", has this been a problem within the last 12 months?
Yes ❒ No ❒ N/A ❒ R/A ❒

• If any problem has been identified in any of the above questions, what would you say is the frequency of this type of situation within the last 12 months?

1. Only once   2. A few times   3. Monthly   4. Weekly

Explain problems mentioned: ______________________________

____

____

____

42. In general, do you ever feel that anyone is after your money?

Yes ❒ No ❒ N/A ❒ R/A ❒

If "Yes", explain: ______________________________

____

____

____

SECTION 7B:
FINANCIAL DEPENDENCY OF SOMEONE ON THE SUBJECT

43. In the past 12 months, has anyone depend on you for money?

Yes ❐ No ❐ Sometimes ❐ N/A ❐ R/A ❐

If "No", go to question 49.

If "Yes", who?

- Spouse / common law / partner ❐
- Son(s) ❐
- Daughter(s) ❐
- Grandchild(ren) ❐
- Niece(s) ❐
- Nephew(s) ❐
- Other: ____________________

- **Does one of the above also manage your finances?** Yes ❐ No ❐ N/A ❐ R/A ❐
- If "Yes", who? ____________________

44. Does that person live with you? Yes ❐ No ❐ N/A ❐ R/A ❐

45. To what degree is that person dependent on you financially?

1. Totally ❐
2. Partially ❐
3. Episodically ❐

Is this? Permanent ❐ Temporary ❐

Explain: (For example: presently unemployed, inadequate revenue, disability, other):

____

____

46. Does this person have any physical or mental health problem (Include illness, handicap, alcohol, gambling or drug addiction, or mental illness?

Yes ❒ No ❒ N/A ❒ R/A ❒

If "Yes", explain: __________

47. Has there ever been a problem regarding finances between you and that person?

Yes ❒ No ❒ N/A ❒ R/A ❒

If "Yes", explain: __________

48. Has this person ever mistreated you whether it was intentional or not?

Yes ❒ No ❒ N/A ❒ R/A ❒

If "Yes", explain: __________

- **Is that problem still going on?** Yes ❒ No ❒ N/A ❒ R/A ❒

Explain: __________

SECTION 8: SUMMARY QUESTIONS TO ASK THE SUBJECT

Interviewer states: ("We are coming near the end of our questions and we just want to go over a few more issue")

49. Has there ever been a time when you have felt scared or threatened by any one close to you?

1. No ❐

2. Yes, already mentioned ❐

3. Yes, not mentioned, explain: ______

______

______

4. If "Yes" to question 49.3, has this been going on within the last 12 months?

Yes ❐ No ❐ N/A ❐ R/A ❐

If "No" to question 49.4, then when did this occur? ______

50. Do you believe that any one you know mistreats you in any way, whether it was intentional or not?

1. No ❐ *(go to question 51)*

2. Yes, already mentioned ❐

3. Yes, not mentioned, explain: ______

______

______

4. If yes to question 50.3, has this been going on within the last 12 months?

Yes ❐ No ❐ N/A ❐ R/A ❐

If "No" to question 50.4, then when did this occur? ______

51. Do you ever feel that anyone close to you is harming you emotionally, physically (such as hitting you or handling you roughly), sexually, financially or neglecting any of your daily needs - whether they are aware of it or not?

1. No ❒ *(go to question 52)*

2. Yes already mentioned ❒

3. Yes, not mentioned, explain: ______

4. If "Yes" to question 51.3, has this been going on within the last 12 months?

Yes ❒ No ❒ N/A ❒ R/A ❒

If "No" to question 51.4, then when did this occur? ______

52. In general, are you satisfied with your relationship with the people that are close to you?

Yes ❒ No ❒ N/A ❒ R/A ❒

53. Is there anything that you would like to add that has not been mentioned before?

Yes ❒ No ❒ N/A ❒ R/A ❒

If "Yes" describe: ______

SECTION 9: QUESTIONS FOR THE EVALUATOR

54. Were you able to interview the subject alone? Yes ❒ No ❒ N/A ❒

If "No", who was present and why? ____

____

55. Do you believe that the subject was being open and honest with you during the evaluation? Yes ❒ No ❒ N/A ❒

If "No", explain: ____

____

56. Was the subject able to fully participate in the interview?

Yes ❒ No ❒ N/A ❒

If "No", explain (For example: difficulty understanding, hard of hearing, not cooperative etc): ____

____

____

57. During the interview, did you observe any of the following affective states in the subject? Check all that apply:

- Aggression ❒
- Anxiety ❒
- Shame ❒
- Depression ❒
- Fear ❒
- Hopelessness ❒
- Anger ❒
- Sadness ❒
- Other: ____

Comment: ____

____

58. Did you observe any signs of abuse, neglect or mistreatment? (For example: subject being poorly kept, house in disorder, no food, smell of urine, any visible and unexplained bruising or other)

Yes ❒ No ❒ N/A ❒

If "Yes", explain: ______________________________

____

____

59. Do you believe that this subject is being abused?

1. Yes ❒

2. No ❒

3. Don't know ❒

Explain your response: ______________________________

____

60. If the answer to question 59 was "Yes", did the subject:

❒ State specifically that he/she was being abused?

❒ Used words to describe the abuse?

Explain: ______________________________

____

____

____

____

61. On a visual analogue scale, how confident are you in finding of:

Psychological abuse

Unlikely 0 ______________________________ 1 Likely

Neglect

Unlikely 0 ______________________________ 1 Likely

Physical abuse

Unlikely 0 ______________________________ 1 Likely

Financial abuse

Unlikely 0 ______________________________ 1 Likely

62. On a visual analogue scale, how confident are you in your overall assessment?

Unconfident 0 ______________________________ 1 Confident

63. What were the signs and symptoms that you observed of psychological abuse, neglect (active or passive) physical abuse or financial abuse?

If applicable, explain:

Psychological: ______________________________

____

Neglect: ______________________________

____

Physical: ______________________________

____

Financial: ______________________________

____

64. Has the subject been able to confirm if they were: N/A 0

Physically or sexually abused Yes ❐ No ❐ Unknown ❐

Explain: ____

____

____

Psychologically abused Yes ❐ No ❐ Unknown ❐

Explain: ____

____

____

Neglected Yes ❐ No ❐ Unknown ❐

Explain: ____

____

____

Financially abused or exploited Yes ❐ No ❐ Unknown ❐

Explain: ____

____

____

65. Is the subject in any immediate danger? Yes ❐ No ❐ Unknown ❐

66. Does the subject need or want to be referred for any help?

Yes ❐ No ❐ Unknown ❐

67. Additional comments:

Signature of Evaluator:

Date written evaluation completed (yy/mm/dd):

Duration of interview (hr: min):

Annex 3: PAHO manual

PART II:

Abuse (Mistreatment) and Neglect (Abandonment)

DIAGNOSTIC AND MANAGEMENT GUIDE I

PANAMERICAN HEALTH ORGANIZATION

Regional Office of the WORLD HEALTH ORGANIZATION

OBJECTIVES

1. Analyze the problem of abuse and mistreatment by taking into account an epidemiological perspective, to take countering actions.
2. Recognize the distinct types of abuse and mistreatment.
3. Describe the associated risk factors.
4. Describe the clinical assessment of the victim and the perpetrator.
5. Describe the initial follow-up strategies.

1 – DEFINITION OF THE PROBLEM

Elder abuse is defined as any type of action, series of actions, or lack of actions, which produce physical or psychological harm, and which is set within a relationship of trust or dependence. Elder abuse may be part of a cycle of family violence; it may be caused by caregivers, or may be the result of a lack of training of social and health institutions, who cannot meet the needs of older persons.

Elder abuse and neglect may take diverse forms:

PHYSICAL ABUSE: to cause harm or injury, to coerce physically, as for example to impede the free movement of an individual without justification. Also included in this category is the sexual abuse of an individual.

PSYCHOLOGICAL ABUSE: to cause psychological harm, as for example causing stress, anxiety, and attacking the dignity of an individual with insults.

ECONOMIC ABUSE: to exploit the goods of a person, fraud, blackmail, as well as theft of money or the property of an individual.

NEGLECT OR ABANDONMENT: negligence or the omission of assisting or aiding an individual who depends on this help, or towards whom there exists a legal or moral obligation. Neglect or abandonment may be intentioned or unintentional.

Intentioned neglect is when a caregiver, due to bad will or irresponsibility, ceases to provide an older person with the help this person may need. Unintentional neglect is when the caregiver does not provide assistance, either due to ignorance or incapacity.

1.1 – Risk Indicators

Elder abuse may be represented through the four categories mentioned, and may manifest itself in different ways (Table 1.1).

Table 1.1 – Manifestations of abuse

Types of physical abuse	
• Shoving • Hitting • Forcing someone to eat or drink something • Forcing someone to be in an inappropriate position • To attach or bind someone • Pinching	• Burning (with cigarettes, fluids...) • Injuries or wounds • Breaking bones • Pulling Hair • Shaking • Putting or throwing food or water at someone • Sexual abuse

Types of psychological or emotional abuse	
• Threaten to abandon someone • Non-justifiable accusations • Harassment • Physical or verbal intimidation • Infantilizing the individual • Limiting the rights of an individual to:	– a private life – take a decision – medical information – vote – receive mail – communicate with others

Types of financial abuse	
• Using the resources of the older person for the benefit of the caregiver • Financial blackmail	• To take possession of the property of an individual • Coercion to sign legal documents, such as wills, acts of property, etc.

Types of neglect or abandonment	
• Neglecting the dehydration of an individual • Neglecting the good nutrition of an individual • Ignoring untreated ulcers	• Neglecting the hygiene of an individual • Not healing open wounds or lesions • Maintaining an unhealthy environment • Abandoning the person in bed, the streets, or a public institution

2 – BASIS OF THE DIAGNOSTIC

2.1 – Risk Factors

IN THE FAMILY:

- Caregiver stress
- Level of dependence of the older person
- History of violence in the family
- Personal and financial difficulties of the caregiver
- Alcoholism or other addictions
- A lack of information and resources concerning the attention required towards a person with incapacities
- Social isolation of the caregiver
- Lack of support and rest for the caregiver, who is responsible for a disabled or incapacitated individual 24 hours per day, seven days per week.

IN THE INSTITUTIONS AND COMMUNITY HOMES:

- The institution prevents or impedes contacts between the older individual and the community.
- This institution is not in an official registry and lacks appropriate accreditation. There is no control or surveillance by public authorities.
- These institutions may hire attendants, nurses or caregivers who lack the proper training to care for people who are fragile and incapacitated.
- It is difficult for the institutions to keep a good and necessary ratio between the staff and the patients, who may be severely incapacitated or suffering from dementia, in order to meet the basic needs of this vulnerable group.
- There may be an overcrowding and a lack of private space for the individuals in the homes.
- There is no evidence that the community participates in the activities of the home.
- The physical structure of the institution is not adapted to the individuals who may be incapacitated and have problems with their mobility.

2.2 – Diagnosis of the problem

The symptoms of abuse and neglect of a frail or dependent older person may take on different forms, and it is recommended that should there be a suspicion of abuse or mistreatment, the doctor undertakes a thorough evaluation of the patient, both through a physical exam and a private interview. Table 1.2 presents the most common indicators of abuse or mistreatment. The critical paths of the diagnosis of the problem are presented in the Diagram 1.1.

Table 1.2 – Indications on the Possibility of Elder Abuse or Neglect[32]

Type	History	Physical exam
Physical abuse	Changes in the description of facts, which are in any case improbable or in conflict with the wounds.	Presence of lesions, especially multiple and with differing levels of deepness and healing. Dehydration or malnutrition. Fractures of undetermined causes. Presence of wounds which were not taken care of. Signs that the individual may have been tied, bound, or hit. Sexually transmissible diseases.
By medication	Frequent medical admissions or consultations due to medication mistakes.	Signs of intoxication due to overmedication, or under-medication.
Psychological abuse	History of conflict between the older person and the family or caregiver.	In general the commentaries and explanations diverge when the caregiver and patient are interviewed separately. It has been observed commentaries on the part of the caregiver which lowers the esteem or infantilizes the older person. It also has been observed that the older person has difficulty speaking in the presence of the caregiver.
Neglect	– Recurring episodes of illness, despite proper education and support. – Untreated medical problems.	Hygiene problems, undernourishment, hypothermia, untreated ulcers, under-medication.

32. Modification of: Yoshikawa TT, Cobbs EL, Brummel-Smith K: Elder Mistreatment: Abuse and Neglect. In: Practical Ambulatory Geriatrics, p. 134, 1998 (2nd Ed.).

Diagram 1.1 – Diagnostic Guideline on Elder Abuse or Neglect[34]

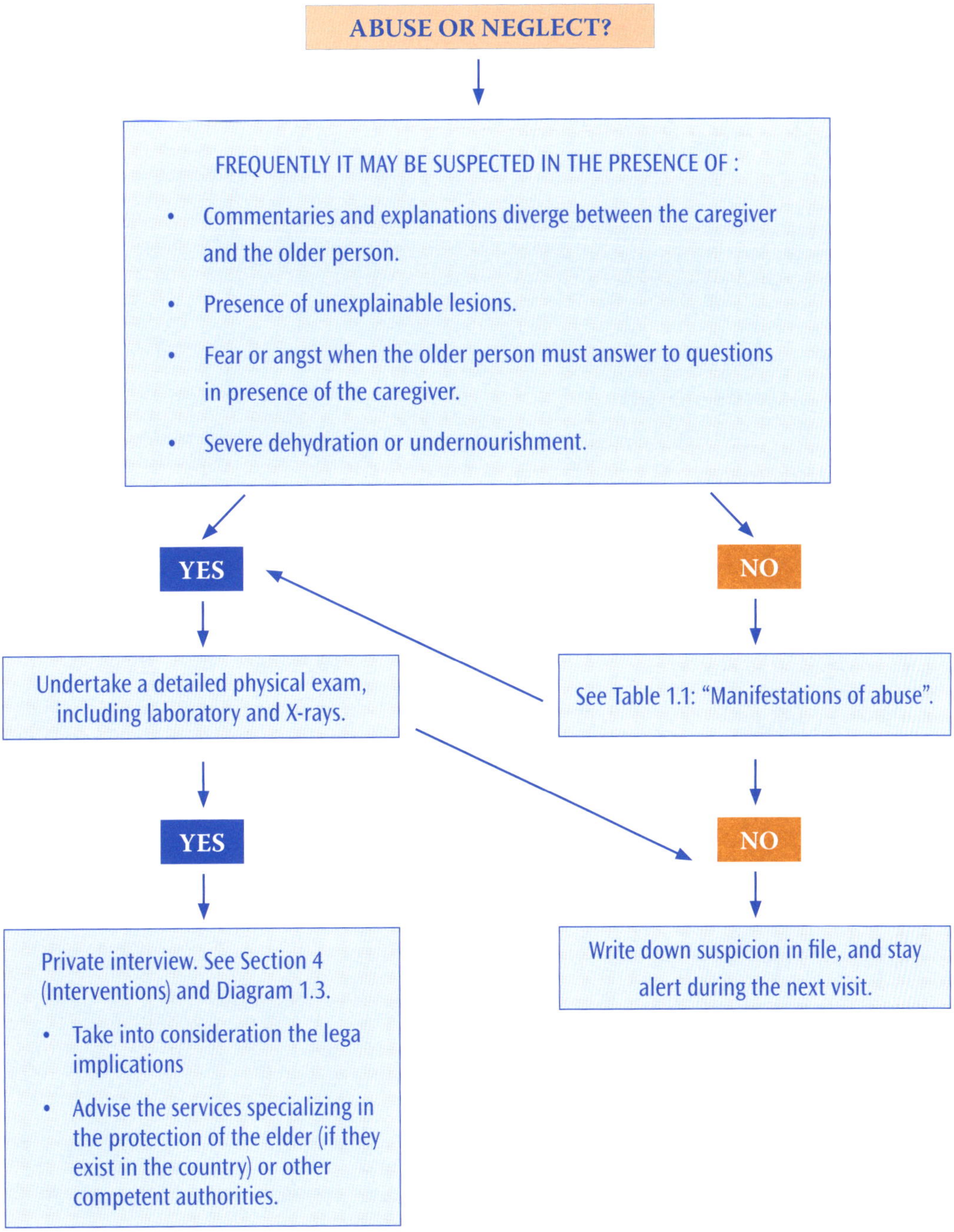

33. Taken from: American Medical Association: Diagnostic and Treatment Guidelines on Elder Abuse and Neglect, p. 13, 1992, Chicago.

3 – BASIS FOR THE TREATMENT OF THE DIAGNOSIS

Diagram 1.2 – Treatment Guideline on Elder Abuse and Neglect[34]

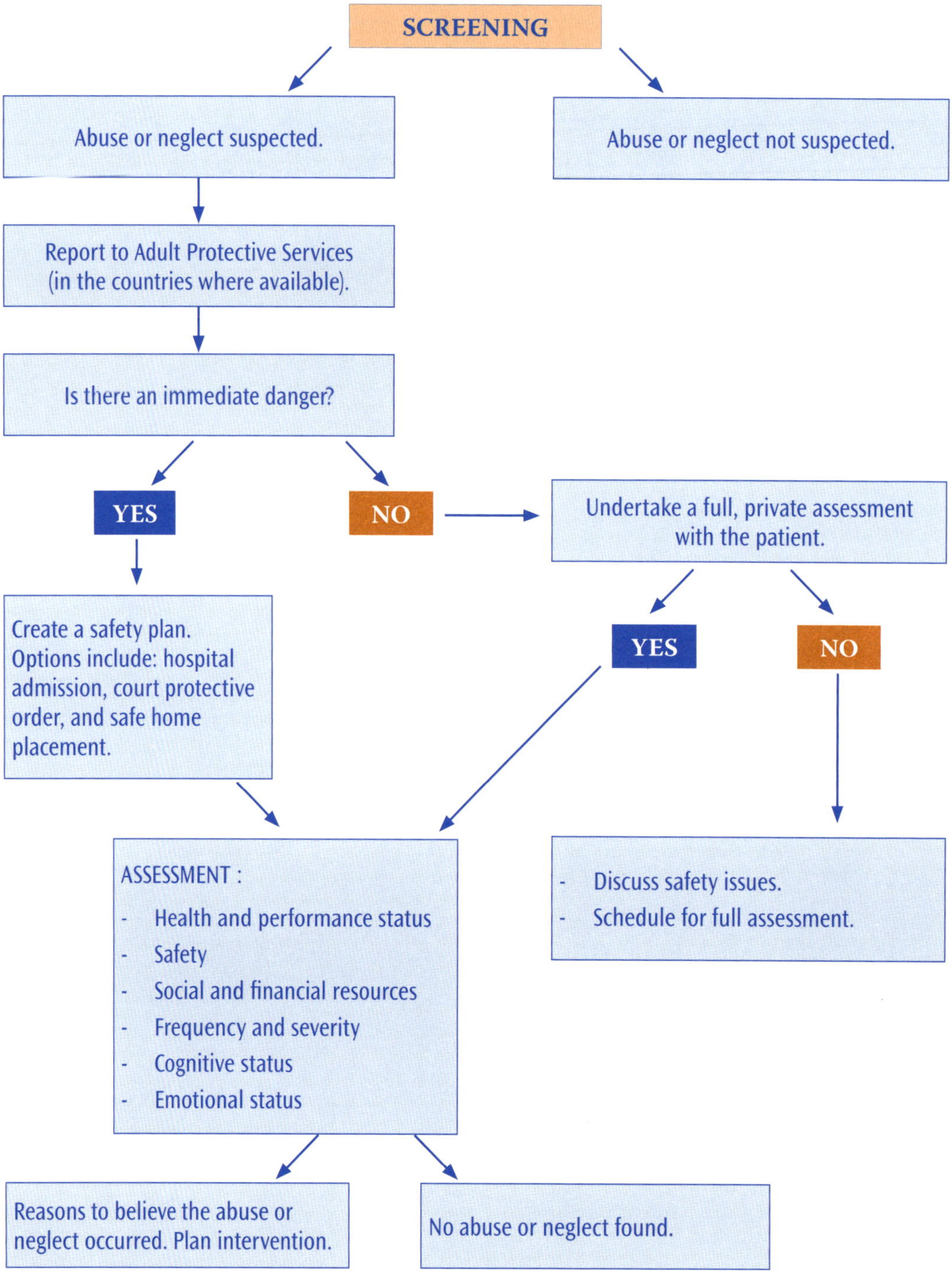

34. Taken from: American Medical Association: Diagnostic and Treatment Guidelines on Elder Abuse and Neglect, p. 13, 1992, Chicago.

3.1 – Intervention Plan

In every case of abuse or neglect, the intervention will depend principally on the acceptance by the older individual of the offer of assistance, as well as the person's capacity to decide. The level of intervention will depend on the services for the protection of the elderly available within the country. We suggest a way to develop a general program in Diagram 1.3, and ask you to decide what path to take in your region.

Diagram 1.3 –Intervention scheme in case of abuse or neglect

INTERVENTIONS

↓

COORDINATE APPROACH WITH ADULT PROTECTIVE SERVICES OR AS MANDATED IN YOUR COUNTRY

PATIENT IS WILLING TO ACCEPT VOLUNTARY SERVICES

- Educate the patient about the incidence of elder abuse and neglect, and the tendency for them to increase in frequency and severity over time.
- Implement a safety plan (ex: safe home, court protective order, hospital admission).
- Provide assistance that will alleviate causes of mistreatment (ex: refer the caregiver to a drug or alcohol rehabilitation clinic, provide education, home health, and/or homemaker services for both caregiver and older person).
- Referral of patient and/or family members to appropriate service (ex: social work, counselling services, legal assistance).

PATIENT IS UNWILLING TO ACCEPT VOLUNTARY SERVICES OR LACKS CAPACITY TO CONSENT

PATIENT WITHOUT THE CAPACITY TO DECIDE

Discuss with appropriate authorities the following services or options:

- Financial management assistance.
- Conservatorship or Guardianship.
- Special court proceedings (ex: orders of protection).

PATIENT WITH THE CAPACITY TO DECIDE

- Educate the patient about the incidence of elder abuse and neglect, and the tendency for them to increase in frequency and severity over time.
- Provide written information on emergency numbers and appropriate referrals.
- Develop and review safety plan.
- Develop a follow-up plan.

4 – KEY POINTS TO REMEMBER

- Abuse and neglect are problems which are little known within the health profession.
- They appear daily during geriatric consultations.
- They happen to older people.
- Psychological and financial abuse, with neglect and abandonment are the most common forms of abuse and mistreatment towards older people.

5 – SUGGESTED READINGS

American Medical Association: Diagnostic and Treatment Guidelines on Elder Abuse and Neglect, 1992, Chicago: AMA.

International Network for the Prevention of Elder Abuse. www.inpea.net

Lachs MS, Pillemer K: Abuse and Neglect of Elderly Persons. NEJM 1995; 332:437-442.

National Center on Elder Abuse. www.elderabusecenter.org

World Health Organization: Missing Voices. Views of Older Persons on Elder Abuse, 2002, WHO/NMH/VIP/02.1. www.who.int/hpr/ageing/elderabuse.htm

Yoshikawa TT, Cobbs EL, Brummel-Smith K: Elder Mistreatment. Abuse and Neglect. In: Practical Ambulatory Geriatrics, p.134, 1998 (2nd. Ed.).

Annex 4: Summaries of country reports

Summary of report from Australia

Focus groups

Focus groups with older people

This report is based on the views of 23 senior people from Victoria, Australia. Three focus group discussions were held, consisting of, respectively, a mixed group of eight males and females, a group of seven females, and a group of eight males. Most of the participants were recruited from three seniors' organizations. Participants' ages ranged from 65 years to 84 years.

A number of general and often related issues emerged from the discussions and are likely to have influenced responses to individual questionnaire items:

- A recurring theme in the mixed group was the participants' awareness of the subtle and not so subtle changes in the way society regarded them as being "less of a person" as they aged.
- It is becoming less likely that older people have a consistent and close relationship with a doctor who knows them well.
- The questions as written come across as somewhat stilted and formal and sometimes are expressed too "clinically".
- Older people's dependency on their carers could prevent open and honest answers regarding abuse.
- Not all general practitioners have the skills to ask the questions in a sensitive way that does not alienate, embarrass or potentially silence an older person.
- Pressures on general practitioners' time and patients' costs were identified as potential problems. Participants thought it unlikely that the 12 questions could be asked in a single visit.
- What are the next steps for general practitioners if they establish a suspicion of abuse? This was thought to be an issue of determining which agency is best placed to support an older person.

The most relevant questions chosen by the groups were Questions 8, 11 and (equally) 4, 5 and 6 (in order of relevance).

Question 4: There was general agreement that this question was important, especially when considered in the context of the whole set of questions. However, participants identified a number of problems with the wording of the question. It was too long and came across as convoluted, principally because the list of examples given is too extensive. General practitioners could choose from the list of examples those that they thought most appropriate. For instance, a general practitioner would not ask about a hearing aid if it was clear that the person did not need one.

The phrase "needed things" sounded clumsy and should be changed to "things you need". Although it was understood that the idea of being "prevented" from doing something was an important indicator of possible abuse, some suggested that it was likely to be very confronting and there may be other ways of encouraging people to open up. The question could be introduced by saying "I'm going to ask you just a few questions about the things you need, such as your food and any medicines you need, your clothing and living space", followed by "Is it easy for you to get all you need in the way of food and medication and so on? Has anyone ever denied you these things?"

A number of suggestions for rewording were made to overcome some of the problems mentioned:

"Has anyone prevented you from having essentials necessary to your well-being?"

"If you needed .../when you need ..., has anyone ever stopped you from getting them?"

It was thought that the second part of the question was important but could be asked more simply, e.g. "Does this happen often?" The question could then be followed up with further questions that encourage people to "tell their own story".

Question 5: The participants' experience was that psychological abuse, intimidation, verbal abuse and bullying, which the question included, often had a profound effect on older people and potentially were very demeaning. Such abuse was difficult to prove, as it could be denied easily, especially if the older person had dementia.

Most thought the question was too wordy and included too many ideas. Some suggested alternatives were:

"How do you get on with your family or the person/people who care for you?" (followed by more specific questions, depending on the response).

"Have you ever been intimidated by the people who are close to you/your family/the person who cares for you?"

Question 6: Participants thought that the ideas embedded in this question were very important for detecting elder abuse. There was consensus that the wording was relatively clear, and all the ideas in the question were important. However, they also thought that there were at least three separate ideas in the question – being taken advantage of, being prevented from doing things, and being patronized or not taken seriously. Each was very important, and putting them together in one question made it difficult to follow.

The forms of psychological abuse referred to in the question are sometimes very difficult to do anything about. Participants talked about their experiences of older people who covered up, denied, forgave or ignored some forms of psychological abuse for various reasons, but frequently because they did not want to lose the relationship they had with the abusing person.

Question 8: This question was regarded as important for detecting elder abuse, particularly as there is considerable potential for financial abuse of older people.

Some argued that the two parts of the question should be separated as they were about different things.

It was stressed that some older people would not admit that they were being taken advantage of or being defrauded, especially by a family member or someone close to them. Pride and fear were very potent motivations for hiding this type of behaviour.

There was a general feeling that the question was inappropriate and needed to be simplified. Asking about the unwanted signing of documents should come first, as it was thought to be less intimidating than the first part of the question. Furthermore, the terms “pressured” and “persuaded against your will” should be used rather than, or as well as, “forced”, as they include more situations in which financial abuse could potentially take place.

The phrase “Has anyone that you would trust” is clumsy. It ought to read “Has anyone you trusted”.

Question 11: Participants thought that direct physical abuse was a very important subject to ask about. However, a number of important issues were raised in relation to the question as written:

- Should the question be asked irrespective of whether there is any evidence for doing so or at least a suspicion of physical abuse?
- Should the question be specific or general?
- Do doctors have the skills to ask this question in ways that will encourage people to be truthful? And do elderly people perceive doctors as understanding and able to handle such matters?
- Should the threat of physical abuse be included in the question, or should it be a separate part of the question?
- The wording needs to be simplified. The phrase “impeded your free movement” is too formal and clinical. An alternative is “restrained you or stopped you from moving freely”.

Other suggestions for rephrasing the question were:

"Have you felt physically threatened by someone? Does this happen often?"

"Has anyone physically hurt you, for example hit you, pushed you or impeded your free movement?"

Questions 1, 2, 7, 9 and 10 were considered to be the least important questions.

The 12 questions considered together: The general feeling was that the 12 questions were comprehensive and covered all of the key areas of elder abuse. Two people suggested that all items should be retained. However, the questions that should be asked depended on the doctor's understanding of the older person and the older person's particular circumstances. It may be possible to combine some questions; for example, Question 4 (being prevented from having access to things essential to health and well-being) could well be related to Question 5 (feeling intimidated; someone making the person feel sad, anxious and fearful).

Some suggestions were made for reordering the questions. It was stressed that psychological abuse and intimidation of older people are likely to be the most common forms of abuse. Therefore, Question 5 should go earlier in the list. It might then set the context for other forms of abuse.

It was emphasized in all groups that there was a need for "real conversations" between general practitioners and their patients, and hence the way in which the questions are asked is very important.

The view was that time constraints and lack of appropriate training would make it difficult for many general practitioners to use the instrument effectively. Nevertheless, general practitioners are at the front line of health care, and there are strong arguments for any initiatives that increase their awareness and understanding of elder abuse. Initial training and ongoing professional development around elder abuse issues would be necessary.

Australia's population is culturally and linguistically diverse. It would, therefore, be necessary to test out the effectiveness of the questions with different cultural groups, including the language used to refer to the various forms of elder abuse.

It is clear that participants favoured wording that was as simple and as straightforward as possible. For this reason, they tended to think that long lists of examples, as in Question 4, should not be included, although they realized that examples were sometimes necessary for clarification. In refining the tool further, it is important to maintain a balance between clarity, simplicity and brevity. In reality, and used effectively, some of the examples in the existing questionnaire could be included as follow-up questions. Moreover, participants also thought that questions that contained more than one idea should be separated.

It was stressed that questions referring to sexual and physical abuse would be confrontational for many older people and, as reported, should not be asked of all people.

Focus groups with PHC professionals

Two focus group discussions were held, one with nurses (seven females) and one with doctors (two females, two males). All the nurses were experienced in dealing with older patients as they were from hospital and nursing services and a university nursing department. The doctors were recruited from a community and private practice and from two large public hospitals.

The six most important questions were considered (mainly by nurses) to be Questions 11, 4, 9, 12 and (equally) 8 and 6 (in order of relevance). Three doctors declined to choose five items as a short questionnaire on the grounds that all areas covered were important, except for Questions 1, 2 and 7.

Question 4: There was general agreement that this question was important. As with the seniors' focus groups, however, the health professionals felt that some older people who have experienced abuse might not answer this question sincerely, for example because they fear the loss of an imperfect caregiver who nevertheless helps them to be largely independent. As with all of these questions, answers depend upon the manner in which the health professional conducts the interview.

Although they felt a list of examples was useful to inform the patient what was meant by "needed things", it was thought this could be done more simply and less threateningly. The phrase "adequate living space" was felt to be too complex and could be omitted.

Participants suggested simplifying the wording of the question "Have you ever felt that you have been prevented from having the things you needed, such as food, medications, glasses or hearing aids?" to "How often do you feel prevented from having the things you need ... ? Would you say 'never', 'sometimes', 'often' or 'almost always'?"

Question 6: Participants found that the issues raised by this question were extremely important in the risk assessment for elder abuse. The question was too complex, however, as it asked about (i) being taken advantage of (which could well mean financially), (ii) being prevented from doing things (or wishes not being taken seriously) and (iii) being socially isolated. The point was also made that sometimes it is life events or health problems that curtail the freedoms and choices of older people (such as advice from family or doctors to cease driving a car), but resentment can still follow. These three issues are all important, but combining them in one question made it difficult to answer. Therefore, the issues should be raised separately. Since there were questions regarding financial abuse later on, the first part of the question concerning being taken advantage of might be dropped in favour of the second and third parts.

The main discussions in both groups centred on simplifying the question or separating it into two main components. There were also thought to be some unnecessary words such as "close to you" and "for your well-being".

Suggestions for rephrasing were:

"Do you feel that someone is stopping you from doing what you want to do?"

"Is anyone stopping you from seeing people you want to see?"

"Can you do what you want to do? Can you see whom you want to see?"

"Are you prevented from doing things that are important to you by someone you know?"

"How often are you prevented from doing things that are important to you by someone you know? Is that 'never', 'sometimes', 'often' or 'almost always'?"

Question 8: Participants thought this question was very important for detecting financial abuse, as it helps to delve into different aspects of financial dependence and abuse. Again, however, the wording was complicated and confusing, and some argued that the two issues in the first part of the question should be treated separately as they were about different things: (i) misuse of money or assets, and (ii) being forced to sign documents. Some suggested splitting the question into two questions, for example:

"Has anyone used or tried to use your money, possessions or property in ways that you did not want?"

"Has anyone (you trust) made you sign documents that you did not understand or did not want to sign?"

"Are you able to access your own money when you need it?"

Since answering "yes" to any of these would indicate suspicion, the doctors again felt the second part of the question (whether the event was isolated event) was unnecessary.

It was mentioned that the wording of this question needed improvement. The phrase "Has anyone that you would trust" seemed rather complicated, and it was felt that perhaps the "trust" element did not matter so much. Someone commented that if the person was stealing from you or misusing your property, you most likely no longer trusted them. Also, a suggested alternative to the word "forced" to sign documents was "made" to sign, as this was less likely to imply a physical coercion.

Question 9: The likelihood of alcohol-induced violence was considered a very important issue, but both groups strongly recommended that illicit drug use should be added. There were also concerns about the intent of the question, because it implied that someone drinking too much alcohol was necessarily a cause for concern. Participants felt that the more important element here was whether or not someone's drinking or drug-taking habits adversely affected the older person. It was also stressed that the perpetrator of substance-induced abuse did not have to live with the older person in order to abuse them, and so the first phrase was redundant.

Some participants were concerned about the effects of addictive gambling, since this is a major issue in Melbourne and can lead to financial, psychological and physical abuse. The consensus was that it would be good to cover all three risk elements – alcohol, illegal drugs and gambling – in this question.

The wording of this question should be more comprehensive. Suggestions made were:

"Do you live with (have contact with) someone who drinks alcohol or uses drugs in ways that cause problems for you?"

"Is there anyone you know who drinks alcohol, uses drugs or gambles in a way that causes problems for you?"

Question 11: This was considered a very important question. There were, however, some concerns about how the question was written. Some doctors felt they would be reluctant to ask this question unless they could observe some physical evidence of abuse or symptoms of anxiety or depression. Important issues of threatened physical abuse and use of chemical restraint were missing from this question.

Participants also noted that this question was somewhat ambiguous because it could include both accidental harm (such as a fall or bruise when transferring someone into a wheelchair or bath) and intentional harm (being intentionally rough or violent).

Research findings were also quoted to the effect that older people feel ashamed and make excuses for relatives' behaviour. The experience of abuse influences how people define their experiences.

On the other hand, visiting nurses had seen instances where older women who have suffered physical abuse for much of their lives then seek retribution in a caregiving role. Dilemmas of this nature could be understood only if the doctor or other health professional knew something about the present domestic circumstances as well as the history of both the patient and the caregiver.

The question was felt to be overly complex and there was some redundancy. The element of "impeded your free movement" was felt to have been covered in Question 6, regarding stopping someone from doing things or being with people. If retained, however, it would need to be rephrased as "restrained you in any way" or "stopped you from moving around" or "locked you in". There were also suggestions for an overall simplification:

"Have you (recently) been physically hurt by someone you have trusted?"

"Has anyone recently hit you, pushed you or stopped you from moving around?"

Question 12: All agreed that this was a very important question. It could be associated with physical abuse, but having it as a separate question was more appropriate.

As with most of the discussed questions, however, a level of trust in the practitioner is needed, and there is the issue of possible cognitive impairment of either the older person or the abuser, or both.

Some of the doctors thought that starting with a time frame such as "Over the past few years" would be helpful in eliminating episodes that occurred decades ago. After a "yes" answer, PHC practitioners would then need to follow up with questions about the duration and severity of any reported sexual abuse.

The doctors did not feel the second part of the question was necessary ("Was this an isolated event or not?"). The fact that any such abuse had taken place would trigger a more extended interview with the patient.

Participants wanted to drop the phrase "to the degree that it upsets you". This was redundant given the term "unwanted". Also, the word "advances" was considered more Australian than "approaches". Nurses also recommended clarifying "touched you" by adding "touched parts of your body", as this would make the sexual context more implicit.

The following alternative was suggested for the Australian context:

"Has anyone touched parts of your body in ways that upset you, or made unwanted sexual advances to you?"

Although sexual abuse is a real and serious issue for older Australians, several of these PHC professional cautioned about untrained people asking such sensitive questions. Thus, both training and appropriate referral services must be available when administering Questions 11 and 12.

The 12 questions considered together: Overall, the key areas of elder abuse were covered, but most questions needed rewording or simplification and some could be excluded.

There were a few issues that were considered to have been missed. These were:

- Risk factors associated with a relative's or caregiver's illicit drug-taking.
- Threatened physical violence – which could be added to Question 11.
- Chemical restraint – giving older people inappropriate medication or too much medication, which ties into Questions 6 and 11.
- Not facilitating the older person's needs (i.e. neglect), as in Question 4.
- Social participation and involvement in decision making via control of autonomy – this could be picked up in Questions 3, 4, 6, 8 and 11.

A number of general issues were raised:

Several nurses felt that administration of the 12 questions by general practitioners would take longer than the standard consultation time (10–15 minutes). Community assessments and care plans are staffed by trained nurses and social workers rather than general practitioners. However, the extra costs to patients and time pressures on doctors were not considered to be impediments by the doctors.

It was stressed that a health professional first needed to determine whether or not there is cognitive deterioration in the older person, which would affect the ability to ask any of these questions directly. A related issue was the ethical application of such a questionnaire. Should it be used only for older patients who have ongoing contact with the same practitioner? Is it dangerous to use the questionnaire in older people who are seen only once, such as in a hospital emergency ward or an outpatient clinic? What are the next steps for medical practitioners and nurses if they establish a suspicion of abuse? Which referral agencies are most appropriate?

Several practitioners were concerned about asking these questions in front of a carer who might be the abuser. A related issue was that carers might be being abused by the older people.

Some of the questions are phrased in the present tense ("Do you ... ?") and some in the past tense ("Has anyone ever ... ?"). Some consistency concerning the time frame would be useful here. Should the main focus be on the present or recent situation rather than on something that may have happened 10 or 20 years ago?

Workshops

Workshop with social workers

All six participants (five females, one male) were experienced social workers, working in urban and suburban public hospitals, local government, health and community services, and dealing with patients aged 65 years and older.

Several participants were concerned that, despite elder abuse being recognized as an important community issue in the past, both government interest and public consciousness of it tends to wax and wane. Others mentioned their awareness of increasing expectations on caregivers and consequent increased caregiver stress.

In addition to the abuse categories given in the definition used within the WHO-CIG project, specific examples of abuse from their social work experience are:

- Decision-making by family members on behalf of older people. This includes, for example, subtle pressure not to sell the family home.
- Use of cultural expectations and accepted ways of doing things to justify taking control and making it "acceptable" to hit or push an older person.
- Fear of abuse can be a potent controlling force, not only when there have been actual threats but also when there is the perception of threat from others.
- Withholding of information, either to punish or to take advantage of an older person.

It appeared that the institutions at which participants worked had policies and/or procedures concerning elder abuse, but the institutional responses were not necessarily standardized, systematic or current. In none of the institutions was training mandatory, although it was thought that in some institutions examples of elder abuse may be included in more general training.

The interventions that social workers can make include enforcing existing legislative provisions depending on the level of support and other resources available.

The SWEF is much more comprehensive and detailed than the assessment tools currently in use in the institutions where the participants work. Overall, the participants' views about the usefulness of the Evaluation Form were mixed. The discussion below first identifies positive aspects of the Form and then discusses problematic aspects.

Participants thought that the Form was very comprehensive and included many of the factors of which social workers need to be aware. It could serve as a very good prompting tool, helping workers to think about indicators of the different areas of potential abuse. In this respect, it would also be a good resource for training purposes. There was general satisfaction with the breadth of the areas covered, and no important questions or sections were missing.

However, social workers thought that the Form would be very difficult to administer. There was a general consensus that the length and comprehensiveness of the Form provided both practical and theoretical difficulties. Older people may not fully understand what is going on, cognitively, emotionally or intellectually. Furthermore, the participants thought that a key problem with the Form was the difficulty of getting honest answers to many of the questions (e.g. Question 51). To be really useful, it would require a solid, trusting relationship with the older person, something that could be built up only over a period of time. For these reasons, various suggestions were made:

- The Form could be used over a number of visits, or over a period of time once trust had been built up.
- The use of the Form should be individualized, depending on the particular circumstances of the older person. Only those parts relevant to the social worker's suspicions, e.g. regarding financial abuse or sexual abuse, should be used.

Social workers raised two broader issues concerned with the Evaluation Form:

- How does the Form relate to an intervention plan? It was suggested that a manual with assessment and intervention information should accompany the Form.
- Problems with over-assessing people. It was pointed out that minimizing the number of assessment tools is encouraged in social work, so that people are not asked the same questions by different people again and again.

Workshop with social workers and PHC professionals

The PAHO workshop group comprised three females and two males. All five participants had experience of working with older people who had been subjected to violence. Their practice environments were quite varied, including a public hospital, community health, aged care facilities, and domestic violence and sexual assault resource centres.

Participants generally agreed with the WHO-CIG definition of elder abuse but felt that effective solutions often needed to focus upon the perpetrator of abuse (relatives/caregivers) rather than only on the older person.

They would add the following abuse categories:

- Abandonment and institutionalization, i.e. used as a threatened or actual means of controlling the older person.
- Family or gendered violence, i.e. the continuation of violence against a woman into older age, usually by a partner or other family member.
- Decision-making by family members on behalf of the older person.
- Financial motivations and family greed.
- Using fear of abuse or abandonment to control.

Hospitals and social work services at which the participants worked were reported to have policies and procedures concerning elder abuse. However, institutional training was not formal, standardized, systematic or compulsory. It was felt that it was largely up to the individual health-care professional to keep up-to-date with these issues and practices. However, the community counsellors' and activists' centres provided specific training in domestic violence and sexual assault to health and community care professionals and to local government departments.

General practitioners in private practices and clinics do not work from manuals or guidelines but assess older patients in a general sense and refer them to social work, aged care assessment and other government or medical geriatric services if there is some suspicion of abuse taking place. It was pointed out, however, that such documents do exist and that all social workers are very aware of them.

Comments on the PAHO manual[35]:

1. Definition of the problem

In the definition section, some additional details would need to be added in order to make the manual fully effective:

- A separate definitional section for sexual abuse.
- Physical abuse should include "forced medical treatments or interventions".

35. Numbers refer to sections in the PAHO manual.

- Emotional abuse could be separated from psychological abuse. Emotional abuse definitions should focus more on the outcomes for the victim, such as anxiety, depression, sadness and loneliness; psychological abuse should also include "limiting the resources of a person (money, housing, etc.)".

2. Basis of the diagnostic

2.1 Risk factors

Under "Risk factors in the family", it was suggested that one main set of factors missing were various types of vulnerability in the older person, such as disability, dementia, illness and frailty. Another was failings in caregiver behaviour, such as lack of responsibility or greed.

Under "Risk factors in institutions and community homes", there were concerns regarding staff/patient ratios, as these were mandated only for medical staff but not for other ancillary staff in accredited facilities. Overcrowding and lack of community and social interactions could also apply.

2.2 Diagnosis of the problem

The general suggestion in the PAHO manual is that "the doctor undertakes a thorough examination of the patient, both through a physical exam and private interview", followed by the detailed "indications" of abuse in Table 1.2. This approach was thought to be largely unworkable, because general practitioners were not considered the "first port of call" for issues of elder abuse, due to their lack of time and training, the nature of their practice settings, and a reluctance to get involved. Contact points would be local government, district nursing and aged care services.

Diagram 1.1: diagnostic guideline on elder abuse or neglect

This "diagnostic guideline" flowchart had a number of limitations and legal problems that would make it largely unworkable in Australia:

- It assumes the older person will have physical symptoms of abuse, which is often not the case.
- It assumes knowledge and history of the patient by a doctor, whereas people often see a range of doctors and visit hospital emergency wards.
- It assumes that a conflictual relationship with the family member/caregiver is evident, which is often not the case.
- There is no mention of cultural differences or a need for a translator to be present.
- There is no procedure whereby doctors must ask permission before touching older patients. This is especially important in cases of the sexual assault of older women.

3. Basis for treatment

Diagram 1.2: treatment guidelines

There were similar reservations about the usefulness of this flowchart:

- They were too medicalized in approach. Using the word "treatment" makes elder abuse sound like a disease, whereas it is a social syndrome with many facets. The focus should be on removing or lessening the harm caused to the older person by the perpetrators of abuse.
- Referrals would be to a hospital or community social work department, aged care assessment team or, in some cases, police or emergency services. Health professionals would not therefore necessarily be involved in court protective orders.
- This was considered to be essentially a crisis model, whereas monitoring and prevention are also important, and, if possible, help via a change of living circumstances for the older person, or the re-education or removal of an abusive caregiver.

Diagram 1.3: intervention

The focus on educating the victim was not felt to be as helpful as referring the perpetrator to rehabilitation, education or corrective services. Also, the preferred terms were a provision of "options" or "assistance", rather than "interventions", as an intervention seemed to remove the agency from the older person.

Apart from the fact that there was no overall adult protective services system, a main issue not addressed adequately in Diagram 1.3 was that of ensuring the victim's safety, particularly for patients who did not have the capacity to decide for themselves about accepting services. It was also stressed that the whole picture and not an isolated event needs to be assessed.

4. Key points to remember

The participants pointed out that elder abuse in all its forms is actually well known within the health profession in Australia. However, due to funding constraints, there are often not enough services to support interventions for both the victim and the perpetrator of elder abuse.

The participants concluded that the PAHO manual was not considered appropriate for use in Australian conditions for the following main reasons:

- Inadequate definition of all forms of abuse – less comprehensive than Victorian usage.
- Rather simplistic medicalized approach focusing too much on physical symptoms.
- It appears to be essentially a "crisis model".
- There are no adult protective services in Australia and no mandatory reporting of elder abuse.
- Australia is well aware of all facets of elder abuse, and health-care professionals do a more comprehensive assessment than what is presented here.
- Often it is not a doctor or nurse who assesses or assists a victim of abuse. Aged care services are networked and complex in Australia.

- It does not advocate the provision for training and resources of health-care practitioners in elder abuse.
- It assumes knowledge and history of the patient by a doctor, whereas people often see a range of doctors and visit hospital emergency wards.
- It assumes that a conflicting relationship with the family member/caregiver is evident, which is often not the case.
- There is no mention of cultural differences or needs for translators to be present.

Summary of report from Brazil

The first studies on elder abuse in Brazil appeared in the late 1990s. In 1997, an investigation was carried out in four Brazilian states (Rio de Janeiro, Minas Gerais, São Paulo and Paraná), replicating an Argentinian study on how older people (aged 60 years and older) view elder abuse. The results showed that the issue was mostly perceived and experienced as societal abuse and abandonment by the families (Machado et al., 1997). Later on, in 1998, surveys were carried out on elder mortality due to external causes (i.e. identified victims of violence). In the state of Rio de Janeiro, for instance, among people aged 60 years and older, violence ranks sixth in the most common causes of mortality, including traffic and transportation accidents for males and falls for females (Souza et al., 1998). Another study on elder morbidity due to violence was carried out in two emergency care hospitals in the city of Rio de Janeiro (Souza et al., 1999). In one month, of the 5151 cases reported, 384 involved people aged 60 years and older. Falls were the main cause for admission, representing some 60% of the total.

In Brazil, there is no published prevalence study on elder abuse, even though data from some Brazilian adult protection services have confirmed the findings above, by verifying reports of complaints about public transportation, accidents and falls on streets, deaths from vehicles running people over and traffic accidents.

High rates of unemployment combined with high divorce rates make many adults return to their parents' homes. Many become their parents' caregivers and depend financially and emotionally on their older parents. The risk of older people being abused increases, especially when the older person is the only source of family income.

The government's failure to provide proper health care services for older people and the lack of social support for older people put a burden on many Brazilian families. As a consequence, women need to work to contribute to the family income but must also take care of dependent older parents.

Considering both the problems faced by older people in Brazilian society and the lack of training facilities in primary health care, there is a clear need for such a survey to be carried out.

Focus groups

There were seven focus groups – four with health-care professionals and three with older people – and two workshops with physicians and social workers. The groups were held in the city of Rio de Janeiro. Inclusion criteria for the older people were being age 65 years or older, being literate and being free of mental impairment. For health professionals, the inclusion criterion was to be working in primary health care. The major obstacle for recruitment was the fact that family health practitioners, who see an average of 20 patients a day, had to be absent from work in order to take part in this study.

Focus groups with older people

A total of 23 older people took part in the discussions. They were split into three groups – one group of seven males, one group of eight females and one mixed group of eight participants. All lived in urban or suburban areas. Portuguese was the first language of 96% of the participants; the remaining 4% spoke Spanish.

Most of the participants could not clearly understand the purpose of this survey. Many thought they had to respond to the 12 questions and therefore could not extrapolate whether each question was important and/or comprehensible. A general comment was that the questions should be phrased in a simple, short and straightforward way. Furthermore, it was mentioned that some questions, such as Questions 1 and 12, require a relationship of trust, otherwise they may not be answered truthfully.

The most important questions selected by the older people were Questions 4, 5 and 7 (equally) and 3 and 6 (equally) (in order of relevance).

Question 3: This question was considered important but too long. Furthermore, the expression "basic daily needs" should be explained in more details, otherwise most older people would not understand it. It could be replaced by "your day-to-day/daily needs and activities", or could it be completed with some examples such as "washing your clothes", "taking a bath or shower" and "preparing meals".

It was suggested that the question was rephrased as follows:

"In your day-to-day/everyday life, do you need anyone to help you?"

Question 4: This question was regarded as self-explanatory, but it should be split because of its length.

Question 5: This question was considered highly relevant, even though it is long and repetitive. The words "sad", "shamed", "fearful", "anxious" and "unhappy" refer to different emotions and cause confusion.

It was suggested that the question was rephrased as follows:

"Has anyone yelled at you or spoken to you in a way you did not like?"

Question 6: Although this question was chosen as one of the five most relevant questions, some participants felt that "being taken advantage of" is normal in the Brazilian context and, therefore, a doctor should not bother asking this question.

An alternative to the question was suggested:

"Do you feel that anyone is taking advantage of you?"

Question 7: The participants felt that this question was one of the most important (in contrast to the PHC professionals, who disputed the relevance of this question), as in the Brazilian context it is often taken for granted that older people contribute to the family income with their money. The expression "financially dependent" should be replaced with "Is there anyone who depends on your money or who needs your money?"

The least important questions were Questions 2, 10 and 12.

Focus groups with PHC professionals

A total of 38 health professionals who worked in PHC settings took part in the study; 28 were physicians and 10 social workers. Of the health professionals, 85% were female and 15% were male. Most lived in urban areas (92%); the remainder lived in the suburbs.

The physicians chose Questions 4, 11, 5, 8, and 12 and 6 (equally) as the most relevant (in order of relevance).

Question 4: This question explains what daily basic needs are. The term "adequate living space" was difficult to understand and could be replaced with "place to live". Regarding the second part of the question, "isolated event" could be simplified with "Did it happen more than once?".

Question 5: This is a very important question that nevertheless needs some simplification. The term "unfairly" should be replaced with "for no reason".

Suggestions for rephrasing this question include the following:

"Has anyone close to you yelled at you or spoken to you in a way you did not like, or made you sad, shamed or afraid?"

"Is there anyone at your home who usually yells at you or loses their patience/temper with you?"

Question 6: This question contains three different aspects and should be rephrased and separated, as all aspects are important: (i) taking advantage of a person, (ii) preventing a person from doing things that are important for their well-being and (iii) interfering with a person being with somebody with whom they would like to be. The term "well-being" should be replaced with "to feel good" or "things you like to do".

Question 8: Most participants felt that the question was relevant and phrased well.

Question 11: In the Brazilian context, the concept of "free movement" is not always feasible. Living in a *favela*[36] often implies (for all habitants, not only older people) restrictions of movement as drug lords and gangs control the community.

The expression "free movement" was considered difficult to understand. Also, the term "physically" should be replaced with, for instance, "Has anyone ever hit you?" or "Has anyone assaulted, hit or pushed you?"

Suggestions to rephrase the whole question include the following:

"Has anyone ever hit you, pushed you or prevented you from going in or out of the house?"

"Has anyone physically assaulted you, for instance hit you, pushed you or prevented you from going out?"

Question 12: This question was considered an important question by physicians but considered less essential by older people. Those who considered it relevant felt that the phrasing should be more straightforward: The older person should be asked directly whether he or she has been sexually abused or harassed. The expression "unwanted approaches" should be avoided. It was suggested that the word "lately" should be included, otherwise the incidence could be related to a younger age.

The participants felt that Questions 2, 3, 7 and 10 could be eliminated.

In a comparative analysis of the results of all groups, Questions 4, 5, 11, 8 and 6 were the most relevant.

Workshops

Workshop with social workers

The attending social workers emphasized their interest in the issue of elder abuse as they face a significant number of cases in their practice. The provision of help does not follow any protocol or established system, and the majority of the participants receive no specific training on elder abuse. They mostly use their professional experience and training from the area of domestic violence (against women and children) and adapt it to their work with older people. Other aggravating factors are the lack of standard tools, difficulties in following up cases, and insufficient engagement on behalf of the government.

36. Brazilian shanty town.

Entry of an older person into the system is almost always through a physician. This makes it more difficult to detect elder abuse due to a lack of awareness among PHC professionals.

Many of the participating social workers see elder abuse as a cultural and social factor, due to the predominant culture of disregard and disrespect towards older people, expressed by flaws in public policies relating to health care, social issues and financial issues.

Culturally specific risk factors for elder abuse in a Brazilian urban area are family members who work in drug dealing. Also, living in a favela increases the level of vulnerability due to the violent environment, caused mainly by drug trafficking. Together with the impediment of free movement, these factors contribute to a higher isolation of older people and prevent action and intervention when there is a suspicion of abuse.

The SWEF was not considered useful for the Brazilian context due to its length. Most of the consultations in the respective facilities and institutions have an established duration. A social work consultation takes a maximum of 30 minutes. Questions 54, 57, 58, 61, 62, 63, 64, 65 and 66 are considered to be important. In order to assess elder abuse, the older person should be asked about living conditions, family dynamics, addictions of any family members, degree of physical and economic dependence of the older person, and social and emotional isolation.

The social workers also commented on the bank of 12 questions and considered Questions 4, 5, 6 and 8 to be the most important.[37]

Workshop with social workers and PHC professionals

The participants considered abuse as a health and social issue, as the two were interconnected. Psychological abuse, neglect and abandonment occur more frequently than physical abuse. Several participants mentioned a connection between culture, education and elder abuse: "One must learn to respect elders."

Although Brazil has adopted the Elderly Act, a law that makes reporting of suspicions or proven cases of elder abuse mandatory, the lack of training and guidelines becomes evident trough the statements of the health professionals. Some stated that they were able to identify physical elder abuse but often did not know how to follow up a suspicion. Although the social workers emphasized the implication of this law (mandating), the physicians were concerned about their own safety.

37. These results are not included in the findings in section 3.2, as the questions were discussed with social workers only in the Brazilian groups.

The participants considered the PAHO manual to be too long but would use it if it were shorter and adjusted to the Brazilian context. As no guidelines are available, this manual could raise awareness among PHC professionals. They concluded that a tool enabling PHC practitioners to identify elder abuse and neglect is extremely important, as it would allow a prompt counteracting intervention worldwide. However, due to the difficult situation of health professionals in Brazil – with the competencies of a family health practitioner different being from those of a primary care practitioner, and the short consultation time – they recommended two different versions of the protocol: one, comprising five questions, to raise the suspicion of abuse and a more comprehensive one to use as a follow-up tool.

Summary of report from Chile

Elder abuse in Chile is a social problem that occurs both in the domestic and the institutional setting. The estimated prevalence rate is 30%.

Focus groups

Focus groups with older people

There were two focus groups with older people, both of which were conducted in the metropolitan region of Santiago. The participants of both groups (group 1: females only, average age 75 years; group 2: males and females, average age 70 years) had a lower middle socioeconomic background.

The older people did not understand the concept of commenting on the questions but shared their experiences regarding every item. It was emphasized that isolation increases the risk of being abused. Belonging to a seniors' group is an important protective factor, not only to avoid isolation but also to share advice and important information on older people's rights.

Common forms of abuse are deprivation of food and the burden of child care. Older people are often obliged to look after their grandchildren. They seldom try to defend themselves because they fear their children may institutionalize them. Children are often the perpetrators in cases of elder abuse.

Focus groups with nurses

The focus groups with PHC professionals consisted of 24 nurses from different services in the metropolitan region. Doctors were asked to join the discussions but were not willing to participate because of time constraints. In the Chilean context, nurses are the PHC professionals who receive older patients when they sign up at a surgery. Nurses are, therefore, the appropriate professional group to involve and address in Chile.

There were two focus groups, each with nine participants; six nurses shared their comments in written form. Before attending the discussion, each of the nurses applied the 12 questions to 10 older patients.

The professionals selected Questions 4, 5, 8, 9 and 11 as the most relevant.

Question 4: This question was considered very relevant. Its wording, however, is not appropriate, since it is too long and needs to be more specific. Terms such as "adequate living space" and "health aids" are too technical. Furthermore, basic needs such as food are mixed up with secondary needs such as hearing aids. To simplify the wording, the question could be rephrased as follows (selection):

"Has anyone denied you food, clothing or housing to live?"

"Do you feel that someone has intentionally denied you basic elements such as clothing and medication?"

Question 5: In order to detect psychological abuse, this question is very important, considering the high frequency of psychological abuse at a family level. The question was considered to be too long and confusing, however. The following suggestions were made to simplify the question:

"Do you feel that someone close to you has verbally abused you?"

"Are you shouted at in your home?"

"Has a family member treated you badly, shouted or raised their voice to you, used swear words or embarrassed you?"

"Has someone close to you spoken to you in a way that upset you?"

Question 8: This question can be combined with Question 6.

Question 9: This question polarized the participants. Some participants thought the question was essential as it tackles alcohol dependence, which is one of the main sources of intrafamilial violence. The other participants considered the question to be very subjective, as different people define alcohol dependence differently: For example, some members of religious organizations may consider drinking any alcohol as wrong, whereas people who are alcohol-dependent may regard drinking large amounts of alcohol as reasonable.

Question 11: This question was thought to be very important as it points to physical abuse. Some alternatives were suggested:

"Has someone hit, pushed or ill-treated you?"

"Has someone hit and/or pushed you at home?"

Questions 2, 6 and 7 can be eliminated.

Conclusions: The questions can serve as a base for an instrument applicable in Chile. However, they must be simplified and shortened, otherwise they may not be understood. It is important, therefore, to use a few examples that help to illustrate the questions and to address in each item only one aspect. Some PHC professionals seem to be familiar only with physical abuse. The questions could, therefore, draw their attention to further abuse categories.

Workshop with social workers

Eight social workers attended the workshop and discussed issues of elder abuse and the SWEF.

In Chile, there are many cases of abandonment reported by the community. Abuse of older people takes place not only within the family but also at a societal level. Older people are the most vulnerable group in society and are often discriminated against and negatively connoted. Older people do not have a strong lobby representing them on the public agenda. Legal regulations and more financial resources could improve their isolated position.

Furthermore, there are neither specific protocols for elder abuse nor any training and evaluation tools offered at the institutions where the participants work.

The Form is considered long but comprehensible and could be used as an assessment tool. The following adaptations were suggested in order to make the Form applicable to the Chilean context. The introductory part (up to Question 19) can be omitted, as this information is available from other sources such as the medical record. Furthermore, some specific sections need some revision:

- Relationship with grandchildren: some older people have 30–40 grandchildren, but it is difficult to refer to all of them.
- Housing categories: add the category of allegados (homeless families living in a home for families).
- Dependence: this section should also take into account that the dependence of older people can lead to abusive behaviour.
- Handling of cases involving cognitively deteriorated older people.

Summary of report from Costa Rica

In 1994, the authorities of the health sector in Costa Rica declared family violence as one of the country's 14 health priorities, defining it as a public health problem. One of the emerging challenges has been to formulate a policy that tackles elder abuse and that increases public awareness regarding this issue. As in many other countries, prevalence data specifically on elder abuse do not exist and have to be extrapolated from research focusing on other topics. In a survey carried out in 1996 (n=328; 67% of people older than 75 years), 4% of the sample were physically abused on a regular basis, 13.8% were suffering from psychological abuse, 5% reported financial abuse and 2.5% were sexual abused (Jiménez Rodríguez, 1998). One of the conclusions of this study was that older people preferred to live alone due to poor relationships between them and their relatives.

Focus groups

Focus groups with older people

There were three focus groups with 33 older people: one group of older women, one group of older men and one mixed group. Participants' ages ranged from 65 years to 90 years. All came from urban and suburban settings.

The five most relevant questions chosen by the groups were Questions 1, 3, 4, 5 and 9.

Question 1: Feeling lonely and isolated are common sensations among older people, as many do not have good relationships with their families. Some older people isolate themselves because they have been mistreated and fear further repressions from the perpetrator. Sometimes, however, it is the family that isolates the older person because they consider him or her to be "useless". Therefore, the participants regard "feeling sad" and "feeling lonely" as good indicators of abuse.

Question 3: This question is relevant for the detection of elder abuse, since dependence is a source of tension and older people often depend on others. However, the "needs" should go beyond the level of "basic" and comprise also a broader range of needed items. The participants also expressed their doubts about the usefulness of the question, because everybody requests some kind of help or support at some point in their life.

Question 4: The participants considered the frequency of the event to be important. The second part of this question is, therefore, indispensable. The prevention of needed things is a kind of abuse that takes place not only in the domestic setting but also in institutions and in public.

The question should be simplified. The term "adequate living space" is not understood well. Moreover, the question should be shortened by abolishing "health aids such as eyeglasses and hearing aids"; "food, medication and clothing" are essential elements.

Question 5: This question was regarded as very useful for detecting psychological and verbal abuse, which, according to the participants, happens often in the family setting. In addition, all kinds of discrimination by institutions, authorities and individuals (e.g. older people being humiliated or not being helped when using public transport) fall into this category.

Question 9: This question is important in the context of Costa Rica, as alcohol dependence is a widespread issue in all social classes. Drug abuse could also be included in this question. The participants associated the issue with physical and verbal abuse. They felt that the question was well formulated and comprehensible and the wording was appropriate.

Overall, the participants thought that the questions were useful for the suspicion of elder abuse.

They concluded that a good and stable family relationship was fundamental in the prevention of loneliness and isolation. However, the majority of the participants preferred living alone, as abuse happens more frequently when sharing living space with their children.

Focus groups with doctors

Four focus group discussions with general practitioners were held, comprising 26 participants (14 females, 12 males) working in urban and suburban settings.

The doctors would include Questions 11, 5, 8, 12 and 4 (in order of relevance) in an instrument with five questions.

Question 4: This question is considered to be very long and to contain too many different elements. An important indicator of abuse is if the older person is prevented from doing something. However, if the children do not have the means or resources to satisfy the necessities of the older parent(s), then this should not be interpreted as abuse. The question can, therefore, be confusing and should be more precise.

Question 5: This question is indispensable for the detection of abuse. The part "Has anyone close to you unfairly yelled at you, or talked to you in ways that you did not like?" already covers psychological abuse; the other elements of the question are less relevant. The final part of the question ("in a way that left you upset for a long time") can be omitted because if abuse takes place, then it does not matter whether the victim was upset for a long or a short period.

Question 8: Although this question is considered long and complicated, it is well outlined and covers not only the relevant areas of material but also the area of spousal abuse. The time horizon should be specified: Is the question referring to the immediate present or to the past? A part asking about the relationship with the perpetrator should be added.

Question 11: This question is very important and relevant for the detection of physical abuse. It is considered to be clear and comprehensible. A difficulty is to determine whether the abuse was intentional or accidental. The frequency of abuse needs further specificity.

The term "hurt" could be replaced with "injured" or "attacked" in order to emphasize the physical aspect of the abuse. The question could be followed by "What is your relationship with this person?"

Question 12: This question is clear and very relevant for the suspicion of sexual abuse, and the participants agreed that it is important to have a question on such abuse. However, they doubted whether the interviewee would answer truthfully a question that tackles such a delicate issue. Furthermore, this question requires a relationship of trust between the doctor and the patient and probably can be asked only after several visits. When asking this question, it is crucial to have follow-up strategies in place to ensure an appropriate referral.

The second part of the question ("Was this an isolated event?") can help to evaluate the person's risk.

The 12 questions considered together:

- The 12 questions are considered useful as the instrument is short and helps in raising awareness.
- To all questions a part could be added asking about the person's relationship with the perpetrator.
- A change of order was not considered to be important.
- The issue of abandonment should be addressed more explicitly in one of the questions.
- Some questions could be combined, for example Questions 5 and 11.
- Since the frequency of abuse plays an important role, categories such as "always", "hardly ever" and "never" could be added to each question.
- It was pointed out that such an instrument could not be applied to cognitively impaired patients. The question was raised of how to handle such cases if there is a suspicion of abuse.
- How should a PHC professional react if there is a suspicion of abuse but the potential victim is not willing to denounce the perpetrator or to be referred for further action?
- Many older people feel uncomfortable when requesting help, either because they want to stay independent or because they are afraid of being rejected. This factor can hamper the detection of abuse.

Workshops

Workshops with social workers

Nine social workers from PHC centres in San José participated in this workshop to evaluate the SWEF and to discuss training and assessment strategies in their workplaces.

Prevailing political and institutional policies do not cover and protect older people. Current economic and social conditions affect them – as a highly vulnerable group – directly. There is a lack of resources and also of supportive networks in the community to tackle the problem of elder abuse. Some institutions and associations carry out very valuable but isolated efforts, centred around the greater metropolitan area. A significant proportion of the older population living in rural settings does not have access to any counselling services.

Regarding the Form, the participants felt that the questions are excellent but the questionnaire as a whole is too extensive. Awareness regarding the issue already exists among the participants, but the very limited number of social workers impedes appropriate follow-up action or intervention. Also, coordination between the different institutions dealing with elder abuse is insufficient.

Workshop with social workers and doctors

The PAHO workshop group comprised nine women and one man, all coming from an urban setting.

None of the workshop participants has received any kind of training. It is, therefore, underlined that there is a need to organize workshops to sensitize not only professionals working in the field but also the community. The majority of participants do not have access to protocols on the evaluation of elder abuse and the physical and psychosocial needs of older people. Some institutions offer manuals with guidelines on intrafamilial violence, but a specific manual on elder abuse is not available. The lack of an appropriate legal framework is evident and makes intervention difficult. An important step would be to offer training facilities for professionals and also to inform older people about their rights. The creation of a network of supportive services is indispensable.

The PAHO manual is a complete summary of concepts already known and is understood as valuable support to increase awareness of elder abuse.

Summary of report from Kenya

Focus groups

In total, six focus groups were held: three groups with older people (one with 10 women, one with 10 men, and one with a mixed group of 11 people) and three groups with PHC professionals. The discussions with older people comprised men and women who reside in a suburban location of the city of Nairobi. They were all from the ethnic group of the Kikuyu and spoke both Kikuyu and Kiswahilli.

The PHC professionals and social workers for both the focus groups and the workshops were selected from the Kenyatta National Hospital. The PHC professionals consisted mainly of dentists[38] who practise at the hospital and teach at the University of Nairobi.

Focus groups with older people

The older people discussed their perceptions and views of elder abuse and its different categories. They also shared their experiences regarding each question but did not comment on the usefulness and the comprehensibility of questions.

Loneliness is a common problem experienced by all participants, owing to the fact that the majority of their children have gone to look for paid employment while grandchildren spend most of their time in school. "Resting on the chin" was identified as an outward expression of loneliness. Since older women experience more isolation than older men, loneliness has a gendered dimension.

Most forms of abuse relate to or originate from the fact that the majority of older people seek assistance from other people. Reciprocal help is part of humanity and is cherished in the traditional African family. However, with ongoing social changes, especially related to urbanization, this idea is now disdained. According to the participants, their seeking for help elicits abuse, disdain, name-calling and emotional abuse.

Abuse of alcohol by close family members, especially sons, is an important source of elder abuse, since the elder parents are usually on the receiving end of their alcohol-dependent sons' poor behaviour and abuse. In most households, the young males are the main or only abusers of the older people.

38. As it was impossible to gather enough general practitioners for the focus groups, dentists were addressed and invited to join the groups of PHC professionals.

The burden of child care on older people is overwhelming. In almost all households, older people take care of the needs of their grandchildren.

Financial insecurity is the most important source of elder abuse; where it exists, it is sufficient to prompt suspicion of elder abuse. The older people have no reliable or known source of income to meet their basic needs. In spite of the financial insecurity older people face, financial dependence on them is very high. The average household has four children or grandchildren fully dependent on elderly people for financial support for food, clothing, fees and medical care.

Most abuse is emotional, which has a far-reaching impact on the older people. Sexual abuse was not identified as an experienced form of elder abuse. The issue of sex is too sensitive in an African context, since it is not a matter to be discussed in public, especially with "strangers".

Close family members are the main abusers of older people. Although older women identify their sons as frequent perpetrators, older men claim their wives and children to be their abusers. At the household level, older people reported the following misconduct and situations that characterize their living situation to warrant suspicion of elder abuse: alcohol-dependent sons, lack of respect for parents, sons projecting their failure on parents, abandoned children, refusal to help in domestic chores and demand for food.

Focus groups with PHC professionals

The three focus groups with physicians chose Questions 4, 5, 1, 8 and 12 to be the most relevant from the bank of 12 questions.

Question 1: Loneliness is considered important in detecting elder abuse because loneliness is a real issue among older members of society today. The question tackles only one issue and therefore is appropriate. It is also a short and easily understandable question without any redundancy.

Question 4: This question is important in detecting elder abuse. The examples provided make the question comprehensible. The question guides the respondent in terms of what is required, and there is no redundancy. The wording is clear and gives the respondent the opportunity to explore.

Question 5: This question is important in detecting elder abuse. The question is too wordy and long-winded, however, to the extent that an older patient may forget the beginning of the question by the time the questioner has finished enquiring. A suggestion for rephrasing is as follows:

"Are there times when a person close to you unfairly treated you? How did you feel? If yes, has it happened once or several times?"

Question 8: This question can be used to detect elder abuse because it is a common phenomenon in modern society. The wording is appropriate and self-explanatory. There is no element of redundancy, and the question can create an environment for discussion with the respondent.

Question 12: Although this question is important in detecting elder abuse, the question was regarded as very controversial. In the African context, sex is a sensitive topic for older people. The question may not be culturally appropriate, since it may cause discomfort. Therefore, the question may not be answered by many older respondents.

A suggested alternative was:

"Has anyone touched you in ways you did not like or made unwanted sexual approaches towards you? If yes, was it once or several times?"

Questions 2, 7 and 11 were the least relevant and could be eliminated.

In the opinion of the PHC professionals, the questions are an important tool in assisting to detect elder abuse. The items cover the most critical aspects that the older people are subject to and experience in everyday social life. Issues of loneliness, dependence on others for their basics, being mistreated, being vulnerable at the hands of the powerful, being taken advantage of, having overwhelming financial responsibility, and being caregivers in their state of fragility are current critical issues that the questions capture.

Workshops

Two workshops were held: one with social workers (nine participants) and another with social workers and PHC professionals (nine participants). The aim was to gather their views on elder abuse as a social and health care issue, and to test the SWEF and the PAHO manual.

Workshop with social workers

The participants agreed that elder abuse is a critical issue in both rural and urban Kenya. The older population has increased tremendously, but older people are a neglected group. NGOs focus mainly on children and youths rather than on older people. For example, homes exist for abused and neglected children, but older people who experience similar problems have no such facilities or support. This implies that elder abuse is not considered a critical issue.

There is a lack of trained personnel to deal with elder issues. The hospital at which the participants work does not have specific policies addressing older people. Routine follow-up is not available, as social work services at this hospital are provided only to inpatients.

There are some categories of elder abuse that occur specifically in the Kenyan context:

- When witchcraft is suspected (e.g. among the Kisii of Kenya), it is always older people, rather than young people, who are accused. Many older people are burnt to death by the public, with or without "evidence".

- There is no access to health-care facilities, and many older people cannot walk long distances.
- Discrimination by health insurance: the National Health Insurance Fund accepts membership only from individuals below the age of 75 years. Furthermore, the Fund demands much higher premiums from older people, thereby locking them out of insurance.

The main causes for elder abuse tend to be economic in nature. This could be due to a lack of savings or because disabilities and needs often strain the finances of their providers, thus leading to neglect. In addition, the emergence of the nuclear family contributes to the loneliness and isolation of older people.

The SWEF was considered to be applicable and appropriate and therefore to be useful. The social workers expressed the need for intervention protocols, specific training, strengthening of their role to advocate for older people's rights, and increased public awareness. The government welfare system for older people should be improved by providing homes, implementing policies in institutions dealing with older people and the law relating to the their welfare, implementing hospital policies that recognize older people as a priority, and training and sensitizing of all professionals about elder abuse.

Workshop with PHC professionals and social workers

A session was conducted involving five social workers and four doctors to discuss intervention possibilities and to review the PAHO manual. Institutional support is required, such as clear policies to be put in place, social workers to be posted in all hospitals, provision of rescue centres for abused older people, sensitization of all staff and training on issues of older people, and a proper diagnosis, including a social history of older patients. Both professional groups acknowledged the importance of the PAHO manual as a guiding tool to assess the psychological needs of older people. The enactment of legislation on older people at the national and institutional level is considered as a crucial factor to guide interventions related to elder abuse.

Elder abuse is both a social work and a health-care issue. Social workers assist abused and neglected older people to find homes for placement. Since relatives tend to dump or abandon older people in hospitals, doctors have to take charge of the abandoned people.

Unlike social workers, who confront the issue of elder abuse in their daily routines, most doctors in Kenya are not aware of the magnitude of elder abuse. The lack of doctors' awareness is attributed to the limited focus on elder issues from training through to work situations. The low number of older people in the total population compared with the number of children also makes the issue not recognized as such. The consensus is that elder abuse is a problem in Kenya, but society is focused more on abuse of children and women and hence the abuses to which older people are subjected go forgotten. Both professional groups believe that the lack of awareness by policy-makers is the main cause of this situation.

The majority of the participants have encountered abused patients but reacted differently. Doctors feel powerless. Even though sometimes doctors refer patients at risk of being abused to social workers, in general they do little. Social workers either interview the abused person and/or look for the available and proper social support system. For both professional groups, there are neither intervention protocols nor follow-up strategies available at the institution at which they work. Therefore, there is a strong feeling that the content and issues in the PAHO manual are appropriate and that the manual can be readily used.

Summary of report from Singapore

Due to historical lack of discussion and understanding of elder abuse in Singapore, the term "elder abuse" has a negative connotation in Singapore and elicits such fear and anxiety even among health-care professionals that there may be a need to look for a replacement term. As Singapore ages, the government has become increasingly concerned that more cases of elder abuse and neglect may surface and a need for common definitions, systems and programmes have to be put in place to address it. Thus, in September 2003, a multidisciplinary team comprising professionals with knowledge in geriatrics, psychiatry, psychology, gero-counselling and social work was established to manage elder abuse cases.

In adopting the WHO-CIG study in Singapore, the country coordinator had to modify some aspects of this study to suit the local context. The following changes were made:

- The questions were translated into Mandarin, as the majority of Singaporeans are Chinese and the majority of the current cohorts of older people in Singapore speak Mandarin and its dialects rather than English.
- In Singapore, an older person is defined as a person aged 60 years and over. The national definition currently stands at age 65 years, but in practice age 60 years is used by frail care programmes. The coordinator therefore followed such a definition.

- The level of awareness among PHC professionals on elder abuse is very low, as ageing is a relatively new issue in Singapore. PHC providers, not recognizing the problem of elder abuse and the need for screening, were maybe reluctant to test the questions or join the focus group discussions. As a result, the study coordinator could organize only two focus group discussions with PHC professionals. The rest of the feedback was given through written responses.

Focus groups

The PHC professionals and the older people chose almost identical sets of questions to be retained in the questionnaire. Both groups also expressed similar feedback and views on most questions.

Focus groups with older people

Four focus groups were conducted with 45 older people. They comprised three combined groups of older men and women and one group of older women only. One combined group was run in Mandarin. The female group consisted of Hokkien[39] speakers. The rest of the groups were conducted in English.

The general consensus among the 45 older people was to retain six rather than five questions. They identified Questions 1, 4, 5, 6, 8 and 11 as the most important in detecting elder abuse.

Question 1: The majority of participants felt that the word "sometimes" could replace the word "usually". Some remarked that the terms "feeling alone by oneself", "isolated" or "neglected" could replace the term "lonely", according to the Singapore context.

Question 4: Although the majority of the older people thought that this was a relevant and useful question, the term "prevented" came across as a poor choice of word, especially in the Asian context. It was suggested that "deprive" would be a better alternative.

Some felt that the question was long-winded and requested simplification of the wording for a better understanding by omitting words such as "health aids" and "hearing aids".

Question 5: The participants thought that this question should be split into sections and sequenced. This would make it easier for an older person to understand what each section entails, since the existing question is too wordy. The term "yelling" was not considered to show abuse. Moreover, the question uses too many adjectives. The participants found no redundancy in the question, but again they urged

39. A dialect group in Singapore.

for better clarity in order to prevent the question from being seen as complicated.

Question 6: Use of phrases such as "Has anyone disallowed you to do things you wanted to do?" or "Has anyone cheated you, or do you feel cheated?" rather than asking "Have you been taken advantage of?" was suggested for better clarity.

The majority of the older people felt strongly that the question was too long. The question would be easier to understand if it was supported by a few examples. Nevertheless, they expressed the need to include the question in the instrument, as it touched on restrictions on one's freedom and actions.

Question 8: Most of the older people felt that this question was important because it discusses financial issues, but there were some shared feelings that it should be divided into two parts. The first part should be focused on "tried to use your money" and the second part on "forced to sign documents". A few of the older people were of the opinion that since the question refers indirectly to family members, it would sound better if the phrase "anyone you trust or close to you tried to use your money" was used instead.

Question 11: This question was considered necessary in order to detect elder abuse. Some concerns were raised about the sensitivity of the question. In an Asian context, older people may not wish to relate their sufferings due to fear of "losing face", especially if physical injuries were inflicted by family members. Suggestions were made to change the word "impede" for a simpler term such as "restricted". Some suggested that the general practitioner should ask this question if they see signs of bruising on an older person. It was pointed out that the second part of the question was needed in order to assess the degree of abuse.

Overall comments on the questions were:

- Emotional abuse of older people needs to be considered in the instrument, and questions should attempt to address that.
- The 12 questions have not addressed the neglect component adequately, but there is a need to do so.
- Questions designed have to be culture-specific and not tailored to suit Western countries, as certain questions are still regarded as too sensitive to ask.

The participants felt that Question 7 could be eliminated.

Focus groups with PHC professionals

Two focus groups were held with 12 general practitioners. In addition, the questions were mailed to general practitioners, of whom eight sent back comments on the questions.

The 20 study participants chose Questions 11, 4, 5, 8 and 3 as the five most relevant (in order of relevance).

Question 3: This question is considered to be rather vague, as it is not clear what aspect of elder abuse it focuses on. There is a need to explain what "basic daily needs" are. The question has a negative connotation, which might put off some older people and force them to deny a potential abuse. Furthermore, this question would be difficult to translate into Mandarin because there is no direct word for "depend".

Some suggestions to rephrase this question included the following:

"Are there disagreements between you and the caregiver?"

"Do you usually need someone to help you with basic daily needs?"

"Who do you depend on most of the time for help with your basic daily living?"

"Are you independent? Or do you need help in basic activities of daily living (ADL)?"

Question 4: This question is essential. Examples should be provided to make it clearer. Too many different aspects are included in this question. Only one focused question should be asked, otherwise it might be confusing. For instance, what is "adequate living space"? How does one define "adequate"? Does "space" refer to the older person's bedroom or to the whole house?

Needed things should be assessed separately, as some are essentials and some are not.

Question 5: This question is long and complex. However, it is a good and direct question, and an important one to use when asking about physical abuse. It was thought that "scolding" was a better word than "yelling", as some older people have difficulty with hearing. There is a need to ask about one emotion at a time ("sad, shameful, fearful, anxious and unhappy"). The second part of the question (asking about frequency) can be omitted.

Some suggestions to rephrase this question included the following:

"Has anyone close to you upset you by yelling at you or scolding you?"

"Has anyone ever shouted at you or said things that hurt your feelings?"

"Has your family or anyone at home shouted at you or scolded you or talked about you in a way that upset you for a long time?" If clarification is needed, ask "make you feel very sad, worried, fearful, ashamed, useless and unhappy".

"Has anyone close to you unfairly yelled at you, or talked to you, or made you feel especially sad, shamed, fearful, worried or unhappy in a way that upset you for a long time?"

"Has anyone close to you yelled at you or been unkind to you?"

Question 8: This was considered a very good question that was relevant and simple. The second part is not required. Some examples for better understanding by an older person (e.g. property, objects, money, possessions, etc.) should be included.

Instead of the phrase "sign documents", the term "thumb print" could be used, as most older people in Singapore have little or no education. Relatives can also be included when one asks an older person about people they would trust.

Some suggestions to rephrase this question included the following:

"Have you been cheated financially by someone you trust?"

"Has anyone asked you to sign away your money and/or your house?"

"Has anyone you trust misused or tried to misuse your money, possessions or property, or forced you to sign documents that you did not understand or did not want to sign?"

Question 11: All general practitioners found this question relevant and important in detecting elder abuse, as it is direct and easy to ask.

A suggestion to rephrase this question was as follows:

"Has anyone physically hurt you, for example hit you, pushed you or locked/tied you up?"

Questions 7, 9, and 11 were considered the least relevant.

By looking at all the questions together, some final comments were made:

- For screening, there should be two prerequisites. One is privacy and the other is reporting of the questions. All these questions should be asked in a more conversational way rather than like a questionnaire or checklist. General practitioners could become very familiar with these questions and it would be then easier to include this as part of their consultation.
- As general practitioners spend on average only 15–20 minutes with a patient, 12 questions are more than enough. General practitioners can also pick up those questions that are relevant to the condition of the older person.
- Asking these questions would also require physical examination as part of the screening.
- Nurses rather than physicians could ask all of these questions.
- General practitioners can ask these questions only after the older person has visited the clinic a few times.
- There might be a need to reorder the questions in order to get a better response. For example, asking Question 1 first might not elicit any response at all, whereas asking Questions 2 and 3 first might elicit a response.
- Older men are more reluctant than women to answer the questions.
- Generally, it was difficult to translate these questions into either Chinese and its dialects or Bahasa Melayu.

Workshops

Workshop with social workers

A workshop was conducted with 18 social workers from different settings, such as hospitals in Singapore and voluntary welfare organizations. The main purpose of the workshop lies in eliciting the social workers' perceptions and views on the applicability of the SWEF in Singapore. Feedback included issues raised on the wording of the Evaluation Form, which was viewed as limiting and not providing ample space for the social worker or doctor doing the assessment to explore further. The social workers expressed their reservations about the usefulness and the length of the Form and thus not being able to focus on assessing the depth of the abuse. For a crisis management or intervention situation such as elder abuse, it would be desirable to narrow down the questions and offer more emphasis to ask questions that analyse the seriousness, history and frequency of the abuse. Furthermore, the participants were unsure about the applicability of the Form to the Singapore context, bearing in mind that it was developed for a non-Asian setting. Questions need to be designed in a manner that takes into consideration the cultural sensitivities specific to the different contexts.

The social workers came to a consensus that elder abuse should be viewed as having different categories and thus each category should be accorded equal importance. This can be done by devising a checklist with risk indicators for detection of each different type of abuse and that point towards therapy and intervention.

Workshop with social workers and PHC professionals

A workshop was organized with ten participants (general practitioners and social workers) to discuss the applicability and relevance of the PAHO manual from the participants' occupational and contextual perspectives.

General practitioners and social workers noted that the definition of elder abuse in the PAHO manual is different from the definition provided by the National Center on Elder Abuse (NCEA). The latter definition comprises seven categories of elder abuse, and sexual abuse stands as a distinct category. Abandonment, neglect and self-neglect are three distinct categories. Due to the multidimensional nature of elder abuse, both the doctors and social workers emphasized the importance of adhering to one definition of elder abuse that is used widely, for example the NCEA definition.

Regarding the risk indicators, general practitioners and social workers stressed that a lot of decisions concerning an older person require the family's consent and consultation in Singapore. This could be attributed largely to the cultural context of Singapore, where familial values take precedence over individual rights and autonomy. The lack of resources tends to put the older person's viewpoint in an unfavourable light and force frontline workers to judge situations from the perspective of the family.

Overall, the risk indicators are useful as a list, but for doctors it would not be adequate to call it a diagnostic guide as the indicators were not specific enough. Greater preference was given to a checklist that could be used at the end of the assessment.

Furthermore, it was suggested that the risk factors identified in Chapter 2.1 should also comprise the following: mental illness, history of long-term conflicted relationships, high care needs, dementia and other behavioural issues that could trigger abuse.

For diagnosis of elder abuse, general practitioners and social workers recommended that Table 1.2 in Chapter 2.2 Diagnosis of the problem should adopt a sociomedical diagnosis. This would entail bringing in a pool of general practitioners and social workers with experience in medicine and social work, respectively, for a team discussion.

Regarding an intervention plan, it was suggested to create a helpline for general practitioners that they could use to make referrals when they suspect cases of elder abuse. The group stressed the lack of appropriate authorities to discuss financial management assistance, guardianship and special court proceedings. Furthermore, the flowchart in Diagram 1.3 was viewed as being slightly rigid.

Different professions see elder abuse differently. Whereas social workers are more willing to be involved and would want to share with each other their experiences in handling and managing elder abuse cases, PHC professionals are more reluctant to be involved, especially in asking all 12 questions, unless they are older. This may stem either from the lack of time that they have with their patients or from the expected role and responsibilities attached to each profession. There is a need to reach out to more PHC professionals in Singapore and to increase their levels of knowledge and awareness on elder abuse.

Having a set of questions in the form of the tested questionnaire is critical. However, general practitioners need to know how they can refer to other professionals, such as social workers, in order to be able to handle and manage suspected cases. There is also a need to review the role of nurses in this process of detecting elder abuse cases. However, there may be ethical considerations in this area, and current Singapore law does not require mandatory reporting.

There is a definite need to translate any instrument into the different languages used in Singapore, otherwise general practitioners and other healthcare professionals may find it difficult to ask older people the questions.

Follow-up strategies for detecting elder abuse cases already exist in Singapore.[40] The strategies involve asking older people suspected of being abused a primary question followed by a secondary question before the necessary intervention is assumed. A framework is being designed to be put in place in 2007 or 2008 that takes on a multidisciplinary approach to tackle cases of elder abuse.

Social workers and general practitioners recommend establishing a continuing platform or forum where frontline workers can share information related to elder abuse and journal updates on research into elder abuse.

In terms of strategy, programmes should focus on raising the level of awareness of PHC professionals and their level of knowledge on where to refer suspected cases of elder abuse. There is also a need to involve the government in this programme in order to build the PHC capacity to deal with elder abuse. Without governmental support, engaging PHC professionals is quite difficult.

Summary of report from Spain

Focus groups

Seven focus groups were held: three with older people and four with PHC professionals. The majority of the groups did not discuss the set of 12 questions but discussed the original EASI.[41] Only two groups of PHC professionals commented on the set of 12 questions.

Focus groups with older people

The three focus group discussions were conducted in different settings: a mixed group of nine males and females in a large city, a group of nine females in a small city, and a group of seven males in a medium-sized city. Participants' ages ranged from 65 years to 75 years.

The older people referred mostly to their own experiences and found it difficult to discuss these questions on an impersonal level. In general, the five questions were understood well and the questionnaire was considered to be clear. Question 4 was thought to be the most comprehensible question, followed by Questions 1 and 2, which were thought to be excessively long, addressing too many different issues and in

40. Offered, for example, by specific agencies such as PAVE (Promoting Alternatives to Violence) and SAGE (Singapore Action Group of Elders) Counselling Centre.

41. See pp. 20-21.

need of further specification. Questions 3 and 5 caused some confusion.

Question 1: This question was felt to be comprehensible but nevertheless ambivalent. Some participants thought they were being asked whether they provided help to somebody, some participants thought the focus was on receiving any kind of help, and some participants thought the question was enquiring about help, such as home help, offered to them from a public institution. The list of items was considered a good summary of older people's basic needs; "going to the doctor" could be added. It was pointed out, however, that basic and secondary needs were combined in the question. The item could, therefore, be divided into two shorter questions.

Question 2: The wording of this question was understood well, but the meaning of the second part of the question "Has this happened more than once?" needed further clarification, as some participants thought that one or two occurrences of this type of prevention could not be regarded as abuse. To simplify the wording, the term "prevented" could be replaced with "denied". There was no redundancy in the question, but some participants considered the question too long and suggested dividing it into several questions.

Question 3: The participants agreed that this question tackled a particularly sensitive issue. Some mentioned that they had felt these feelings (threatened and shamed) not only in the past 12 months but also throughout their lives. Furthermore, it was stressed that there was a significant difference between feeling "threatened" and feeling "shamed". The term "shame" seemed to signify a feeling of being embarrassed and should not automatically be connoted with abuse. It might be more accurate to replace "shamed" with "humiliated". A threat can be imposed on a person without previous actions and points more clearly to abuse. Once again, the question could be divided in order to ask separately about these two different issues. An important issue that could be included in this question is infantilization.

Question 4: This question was regarded as being very clear, addressing a frequent type of abuse. The word "force" was felt to be very strong and could be replaced with "manipulate".

Question 5: The participants were unclear whether this question referred to physical or sexual abuse. The word "touched" was not necessarily associated with sexual abuse. Both issues were very delicate and taboo for individuals over the age of 65 years. Nevertheless, a clear separation between these two types of abuse could help to elicit more accurate responses. It was stressed that an honest answer to this question would depend very much on the level of confidence between the doctor and the patient and on the doctor's ability to ask the question in a sensitive way.

Focus groups with PHC professionals (EASI questions)

There were four focus groups, with a total of 30 general practitioners, in four different Spanish cities (Madrid, Málaga, Vilanova y la Géltru and Badajoz).

On the whole, the general practitioners found the questionnaire to be a very useful tool for physicians who did not know how to approach the issue of elder abuse. However, it was felt to be crucial to provide the PHC professionals with a clear definition of elder abuse or with a small introduction, since some participants did not understand the objective of the tool – that is, to raise awareness and to generate a sufficient level of suspicion for elder abuse. It was also unclear to whom the questionnaire referred. Some thought the terms "people", "anyone" and "someone" were too vague; others regarded this openness as an opportunity to obtain an answer without forcing the older person to accuse somebody directly. There was no consensus on the length of the questions. For example, some felt that longer questions were more difficult to understand but would allow for a shorter questionnaire, but others felt that shorter questions might be more comprehensible but would result in a longer questionnaire. The rationale was that the more extensive the questionnaire – even if the questions are made shorter – the more likely that an older person would lose attention. Participants requested further clarification on the best place to administer the questionnaire, since PHC settings are normally busy and leave the PHC professional a limited amount of time for each patient; during home visits, however, there is a risk that other people, including the abuser, may be present.

Question 1: This initial question was considered to be an "ice-breaker" and a general question to detect a potential dependence, an important risk factor for the occurrence of elder abuse. Some thought that the amount of help a person needed did not necessarily indicate an abusive situation. The question was, therefore, found to be of medium relevance.

It was pointed out by some participants that the term "people" should be specified further, but others saw this ambiguity as an opportunity to answer without making a personal reference.

A separation of the question into two parts (basic and secondary needs) might be useful. Activities that were felt to be less important were "shopping" and "banking"; however, "going to the toilet" could be added.

In order to shorten the question, the following alternatives were suggested:

"Do you need help with something?"

"Do you need help?"

"Do you need help with the basic activities of daily living such as bathing, dressing, eating? And with ...[secondary needs]?"

"Has anyone close to you helped you with bathing or dressing? Has anyone helped you with shopping or banking?"

Question 2: The words used in this question were regarded as clear, but to simplify the question it was suggested to replace "prevented" with "impeded". Acts of omission and commission should not be put together in one item. The combination of different circumstances (social isolation and access to basic needs) complicated the question.

The second part of the question ("Has this happened more than once?") caused some debate, as "more than once" was not considered concrete enough.

Question 3: The participants felt that this question was essential in order to reveal psychological abuse. Asking about the frequency of occurrence was considered quite important in this question; the second part of the question should, therefore, be retained. The question as a whole seemed vague, as the group of people to whom the question referred (e.g. close people, neighbours, strangers) should be specified.

In order to shorten the question, a number of suggestions for rewording were made:

"Have you felt annoyed because someone treated you in a way?"

"Has anyone made you feel embarrassed or threatened?"

"Has anyone treated you in a way that made you feel embarrassed or threatened?"

"Did anyone treat you in a way that made you feel embarrassed or threatened?"

Question 4: This question was understood well and regarded as very important, especially when taking into account the high frequency of economic abuse among older people. As with other questions, the second part ("Has this happened more than once?") could be omitted.

Question 5: According to the participants, this question had the highest relevance because it asks about physical and sexual abuse. However, the phrase "touched you in ways that you did not want" could cause discomfort and embarrass both the older person and the physician. Others commented that the question comprised too many different issues, such as threat, physical harm, sexual abuse and feeling frightened. Therefore, it could be useful to divide the question into two parts. One part could ask about physical abuse and the other about sexual aspects of abuse.

The following alternatives were suggested:

"Has anyone threatened, frightened or harmed you physically?"

"Has anyone touched you in a way you didn't like? Has anyone harmed you physically?"

"Have you felt physically or sexually threatened on any occasion?"

A number of alternatives comprised the explicit inclusion of sexual abuse:

"Has anyone harmed you physically? Has anyone tried to sexually abuse you?"

"Have you felt physically or sexually threatened on any occasion?"

"Has anyone hit, threatened or frightened you physically? Has anyone sexually abused you or tried to abuse you?"

Focus groups with PHC professionals (bank of 12 questions)

Two groups discussed the bank of 12 questions. One group chose the five most relevant questions: Questions 3, 4, 5, 8 and 11.

The questionnaire with 12 items was considered too long, making it difficult to retain an older person's attention. Question 1 was thought to be redundant. Several questions could be combined into one, for example Questions 2 and 3, and Questions 6, 7 and 8 referred to the same question asking about a person's personal autonomy and could therefore be combined. A similar debate arose for the last two questions. Although these questions tackled two different categories of abuse (sexual and physical abuse), older people might be more reluctant to answer a question about sexual abuse when such a question was posed more directly.

Some felt that the style of the questionnaire was too Anglo-Saxon and viewed the phrasing as inappropriate. The time frame should be specified further. Moreover, the term "basic daily needs" (Question 3) required further clarification. Question 4 was not precise enough, as it was not clear whether the phrase "Has anyone prevented you from" referred to a person or an abstract body (for example, the community). Question 5 contained too many different adjectives that described different states of moods and feelings. Before administering the questionnaire, previous instructions and information must be given to both the physician and the older person.

Workshops

Workshop with social workers

Ten female social workers, chosen randomly from various health centres in the municipality of Madrid, participated in this workshop to discuss the SWEF and further issues related to elder abuse. The Form was sent to them a week in advance to familiarize them with its content.

The social workers' clientele comprised mostly immigrants and older people covering all ranges of socioeconomic backgrounds. None of the social workers had previously worked in the area of elder abuse, but they had received training and information on child abuse and gender-based violence.

The participants mentioned the absence of specific protocols and guidelines concerning the prevention, assessment and intervention of elder abuse. PHC professionals who referred abuse cases to social workers did so because they were sensitized and motivated and not because they felt obliged to act according to guidelines. A significant shortfall they pointed out was the lack of coordination between social workers and other professionals working in the same institution. Interprofessional coordination was considered to be the key to intervention, which was often too slow and accelerated only if the case of abuse was related to gender-based violence. Some social workers went only once a week to a health centre to exchange information and coordination and ultimately to strengthen the teamwork between the different professional groups dealing with elder abuse. The creation of a round table for older people could offer an important platform for the different stakeholders together to share experiences, disseminate information and offer solutions.

The application of the SWEF was considered inappropriate in the Spanish context because of its length. The average consultation time a social worker had with a client was 40 minutes. The participants also believed that it was rather difficult for an older person to focus on answering questions during approximately 66 minutes. A possible solution could be to administer the Form during several sessions instead of only one session. Apart from the time issue, there were also linguistic problems with the Form, as the literal translation from English into Spanish (e.g. of the term "sponsorship") caused confusion. Some sections were thought to be unclear, such as that on housing (e.g. together putting housing types and characteristics). Two aspects that were not taken into account adequately were (i) the important role of informal networks of older people who did not have a family and (ii) the impact of disputes or problems between the older person and his or her relatives throughout the older person's life. It was criticized further that the Form could raise the hopes of older people, which ultimately could not be met since it asked about issues that were not under the competence of a social worker. In general, the Form was thought to be too direct and negative. In Spain, questionnaires tackling such a sensitive issue used more indirect questions. For example, asking older people whether there were any problems in their relationship with their children was a question that could not be asked. A questionnaire with this type of question should be administered by nurses, as they have more regular contact with patients. The best place where the interview could be conducted was not necessarily the older person's home but rather the health centre or a neutral environment.

It was stressed by the participants, however, that the mere existence of such a Form was positive, as a similar assessment tool did not exist. The Form could serve as a basis for more appropriate evaluation techniques in the Spanish context. The administration of such a form by social workers would also assign them with a role they currently do not have in the assessment of elder abuse in PHC settings.

Workshop with PHC professionals and social workers

The PAHO workshop group comprised five social workers and five primary care doctors, all coming from the metropolitan area of Madrid.

The participants considered elder abuse as a social and health problem that could have very different causes and consequences. However, it is rarely addressed in the institutions at which the participants work. One of the main obstacles for doctors is the very limited amount of time they can dedicate to a patient. They often intervene only in extreme abuse cases. Furthermore, they are rarely familiar with a patient's living conditions, since home visits by doctors are not common. The social workers reiterated that it is not the institution but the individual professionals who show an interest in the issue of elder abuse. Professionals are familiar with the issue, either through other abuse types, such as violence against children and women, or because they have encountered some cases in their consulting room.

The main difficulties mentioned by the participants in the assessment of elder abuse are a lack of the following:

- specific training on elder abuse;
- interprofessional communication;
- level of awareness and sensitization;
- protocols for homogeneous interventions;
- specific definitions and terminology;
- social support for the caregiver;
- circulation of information regarding the existing institutional resources;
- general resources to tackle the issue.

For the assessment of elder abuse, social workers use strategies they know from other fields of work, for example risk factors analysis, and knowledge of the patient's social history and family background. Since they do not have access to patients' social history forms in hospitals, they miss information that may be useful for the detection of potential cases. PHC professionals are probably in a better situation to get an idea of the patient's home and family situation as they often see the whole family in their consultation. The doctors pointed out that intervention strategies must be accompanied by training. It was also stressed that the decision-making capacity of an older person has to be considered. In order to counteract elder abuse, the participants felt that social workers could apply intervention methods they know from abuse directed at other groups (gender, child), and doctors could focus on prevention and raising suspicion. The doctor sees the patient on a probably more frequent and personal level than the social worker. It was emphasized that the most complicated phase in the assessment process is the intervention, as it can have drastic impact on the equilibrium of the family in which the older person lives.

The Spanish Society of Geriatrics and Gerontology and the Ministry of Social Welfare and Labour have published an action guide that includes elder abuse issues (Moya & Gutiérrez, 2005). Since this guide was published only recently, it has not been circulated sufficiently among PHC professionals. The participants felt that this publication is more appropriate than the PAHO manual for the Spanish context, mainly because of linguistic reasons (the PAHO manual uses mostly Latin American and Anglo-Saxon terms instead of Spanish vocabulary), the form of the manual's content (its tables and diagrams are difficult to manage and too schematic), the lack of precision (for example, in the definitions section, the role of the caregiver), the missing emphasis on institutional abuse (the PAHO manual tackles mainly domestic abuse but neglects institutional abuse), and the intervention possibilities (actions suggested in the PAHO manual seem to aim merely at emergency situations and do not include non-dependent older people). However, the PAHO manual could serve as a good basis, but it needs to be adapted to the specific country context.

Summary of report from Switzerland

Focus group discussions

Focus group discussion with older people

One focus group discussion was conducted with 29 older people (19 female, 10 male). Participants had a median age of 79 years.

The general consensus among the participants was to retain Questions 4, 5, 6, 8 and 11.

Question 4: The majority of the older people felt that this was a relevant and useful question.

Question 5: The participants found no redundancy in this question but considered it to be too complicated.

Question 6: This question was thought to be too long. It would be more comprehensible if the question was supported by a few examples.

Question 8: Most of the older people felt that this question was important.

Question 11: This question was regarded as necessary in order to detect elder abuse. The older people felt that the second part of the question was needed in order to assess the degree of abuse.

Focus group discussion with medical doctors

A focus group discussion was held with 11 general practitioners (five male, six female). Participants ranged in age from 34 years to 65 years.

The five most important questions were considered to be Questions 4, 5, 6, 8 and 11.

Question 4: This question was considered to be essential.

Question 5: This question was regarded important to determine whether there is physical abuse, as the question was direct and could elicit a direct response. However, it was felt that the question was very long and complex.

Question 8: This was considered to be a very good, relevant and simple question. However, the question could be shortened or rephrased. The second part was not required. Some examples (e.g. property, objects, money, possessions) should be included to help older people better understand the question.

Question 11: This was thought to be a direct question that was very easy to ask. All medical doctors found this question relevant and important in detecting elder abuse.

Workshops

Workshop with nurses, assistant nurses and social workers

A workshop was conducted with ten nurses, assistant nurses and social workers (all female, age range 26–65 years) from different settings and services in Geneva. The main purpose of the workshop lay in eliciting the nurses and social workers' perceptions and views on the applicability of the SWEF. They also discussed the set of 12 questions and chose Questions 4, 5, 6, 8 and 11 as the most relevant.

Nurses, assistant nurses and social workers raised concerns on how to define elder abuse. The social workers felt uncertain about how to identify a suspect of elder abuse and how to confirm it.

The group was concerned about the level of intervention: How much intervention is required, especially if the older person has a medical condition such as cognitive impairment or high care needs? It was also emphasized that older people with some disabilities should be included. The group stressed the need to adopt multidisciplinary and multilevel assessment methods. Furthermore, it was mentioned that elder abuse and neglect should be viewed as different categories, and each category should be accorded equal importance.

Issues were raised on the wording of the Form, which was viewed as limiting and not providing ample space for the nurse, assistant nurse, social worker or doctor to explore further. In general, the participants expressed their reservations about the applicability of the SWEF to the Geneva context.

Follow-up strategies for detecting elder abuse and neglect are currently being designed in collaboration with the Alter Ego association. They are based on a multidisciplinary approach to tackle elder abuse and neglect. The need to review the role of nurses in the process of detecting elder abuse and neglect was also emphasized. The groups recommend establishing a continuing platform or forum and a helpline, such as ALMA in France, where frontline workers can share and obtain information related to elder abuse and neglect.

Other ideas included the integration of these questions in clinical ethics, geriatric and gerontological curricula. The questionnaire could be also added to the Vieillir en Liberté Internet platform, a programme of community-based health care for older people, centred on respect for human rights, autonomy and solidarity.